Sally's in the Kitchen

by Sally Miller

illustrations by Dave Meszaros
Diane Beeny
and Emily Schaefer

Synergy Press

2009

published by: Synergy Press
                  POB 8
                  Flemington NJ 08822
                  908.782.7101

ISBN: 0-9758581-6-5

Printed in the USA

Thanks to Katie Colosimo for her assistance in helping to prepare the manuscript, especially for taking all those little scribbled notes and making them coherent. I also want to thank Frank Magalhães for his help with typesetting problems.

Appreciation to food testers Arnie, Brice, Dave M, and Katie.

Food prep: Arnie, Brian, Brice, Dave M, Katie, and Scott.

Food tasters: Adam, Anthony, Arnie, Brian, Brice, Dave, Dave M, Don, Gary, Jan, Jerry, Katie, Martha, Michael, Mick, Piera, Rick, Scott, Shen, Shiva, Steve J, Steven, Suellen, and others at Boxelder Basin Wellness Retreat & the Central Jersey Vegetarian Group.

Fact checking was facilitated by the Research Department of the Hunterdon County Library, Flemington NJ and Answers.com, the world's greatest *encyclodictionalmanacapedia*.

Much thanks to the Mid Ohio Laser Engrave company in Caledonia OH for the use of their clip art, to Dave Meszaros for stepping in to help with the artwork, and to Jerry Avins for the cover photo.

Dedicated to my sister

Martha

who through the snows and floods of Fargo
took the time to clip recipes,
make suggestions,
and even argue with me
about recipes, ingredients,
and preparation methods.

And to my friend Brice,
who let me feed him,
first with Stouffers in the 1980's,
later with all the recipes in this book —
he even learned how to cook some of them
himself.

Contents

1. Summer   June, July, and August   Pages 1 - 27

I've started out with some old family recipes which signify to me the start of summer, plus some cold salads and other picnic food. When the harvest of tomatoes, squash, and cucumbers begins in mid to late July, bruschetta, pico de gallo, pickles, and other garden goodies appear. Finally, I have freezing tomatoes and other late summer activities.

2. Fall   September, October, November   Pages 29 - 55

Fall is the time to use up your summer's endeavors by creating hot soups and stews that will last into spring, and to use produce in season, cool weather crops like potatoes, cabbage, broccoli, yams. Recipes are included to warm up the evening (and morning) before the heat is on. More food to make and freeze for less energetic times can be found in the last section of the book, the Fifth Season.

3. Winter   December, January, February   Pages 57 - 89

I have included here oven dishes, casseroles, and other kitchen-warming foods, some utilizing foods you have frozen. You will also find sweets and various holiday treats from a variety of cultures, including Jewish, Christian, Italian, Thai, Chinese, and German, as well as more of my family favorites.

4. Spring   March, April, May   Pages 91 - 121

Included here are some foods that give us a boost after the months of less physical activity — asparagus, berries, stir-fries, chilis, and curries, plus some spring holiday fare including Irish, Christian, Indian, Thai, and Mexican.

5. Fifth Season   Anytime   Pages 123 - 162

Imagine my surprise and dismay after finishing the first four sections of this book to find a large folder from 2001 and 2002 with recipes I had cooked, written down, and tested several times. Rather than try and change the original format, which was already typeset, I got Katie busy again. We have included the recipes here, in the Fifth Season Appendix. Dip into these whenever you are looking for something different, or you're bored, and use this section to stimulate your taste buds and your imagination. They are arranged by Groupings rather than by months. I meant for you to read the book cover-to-cover anyway, so this will help get you thinking a different way about food! The bulk of the recipes are stir-fries and bean dishes, but there are some desserts, menus, and other interesting items.

Fifth Season Contents (continued)

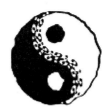

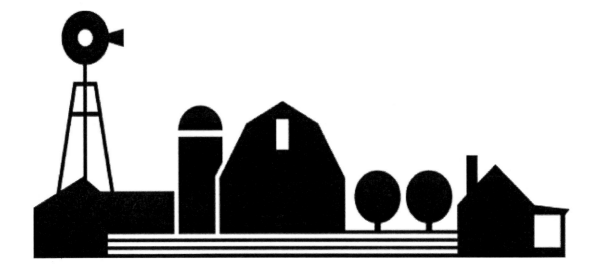

Foreword

Following Sally's remarkable and full recovery from stage 3 ovarian cancer over 13 years ago, without the "help" of standard and accepted medical treatments, I began to realize the great importance of eating foods of high nutritive value. Pouring through nutrition books, I concentrated on jamming as many nutrients into my body as I could with little regard for taste or aesthetics, culminating in my frequent consumption of a blended drink someone once described as "swamp water." But these practices took a toll, psychologically and spiritually.

I began to realize that there are other powerful factors that contribute to your overall health and longevity, namely, the level of comfort and happiness and satisfaction in your day-to-day life.

I have come to the realization that your RELATIONSHIP with your food may be as important as the nutritive content.

My current bottom line is this: if you feel good about your food when you are eating it, and you're still feeling good in an hour or two, and still feeling good the next morning, and still feeling good the next week, and still feeling good the next year, then your food is probably serving you well, whatever it is.

Hard for an amateur nutritionist to say, but probably true. I think Sally has, independently, come to the same conclusion, as this second cookbook includes many "comfort" foods that she studiously avoided including in her first cookbook.

Know your food, love your food, take some time with your food. Consider resisting the temptation to swallow whatever you find conveniently pre-prepared for you on the supermarket shelves or on the menu at the local chain restaurant. That's what this cookbook is all about.

Brice Bock

May 2009

Introduction

I started collecting and testing recipes for this book in 2001, after finishing *Good Eats at Sally's*. *Good Eats* contains nutrition information and recipes that I used during my first five years post ovarian cancer.

This book strays from a stricter vegetarian diet and includes many old family recipes which are almost all high in meat, fat, and sugar. Of course, this explains the heart disease and Alzheimer's and cancer in my family. A diet with meat as a featured member of every evening meal (except 3x a year — when we had strawberry shortcake, apple dumplings, or peach cobbler, all sweet deserts that our family had as a full meal) *could* have given us all colon cancer.

But there was evidently just enough balance in my diet during both my childhood growing-up years and my married years. Though not particularly healthy, I wasn't in immediate need of serious medical care/ hospitalization.

During my single years 1976-1996, however, I tipped the toxicity scale from both diet and other environmental toxins, such as the wood preservative which I soaked wood shingles in up to my elbows for nigh onto three days, or the pesticides in a recently sprayed but still flea-infested apartment (I even wore flea collars around my ankles). I was unaware about this kind of toxins, as well as ignorant of the havoc certain foods have on our bodies. Also, during that pre-cancer time, I smoked Pall Malls (and did so for thirty years before I quit in 1986); drank hard liquor like Yukon Jack, bourbon, and gin; and experimented with a variety of drugs.

It was only after the large ovarian tumor was removed in 1996 that I began to consider what I put in my body. Since then I have learned to enjoy the bountiful colorful world of fruits and vegetables, while at the same time trying to keep a lid on the fats, cheeses, meats, and sweets that my mind sometimes craves.

This cookbook is a window into my diet for the past seven or eight years. Menus of events I've organized are interspersed, including several Celebration of Life happenings to mark off years since my ovarian cancer came and went. I've also included short discussions of nutrition, shopping lists, and information pertinent to healthier eating. It is a constant struggle for me to eat well, and I need to remind myself, as well as others, good ways to do this.

On a brighter side, I'm still cancer free after almost thirteen years. I have finally learned how to balance my wants with my needs. I hope you will enjoy the healthy food I have been preparing and enjoying over the past years, as well as an occasional "bad" food from my past, which I also fix from time to time. This book reflects my efforts to stay healthy, which I have somehow managed to do, according to my doctor Antonia Mattei. I turn 70 this spring.

Sally S. Miller

May 2009

A Note about Using this Book

Although I have divided these recipes into seasons because it seemed the most logical to me, I suggest the first time through you go front to back, stopping to read if a recipe sounds interesting to you, no matter what the season. I hope to inspire you to think about food in a different way.

Different recipes seemed to call for different formats. Though I personally prefer Irma Rombauer's *Joy of Cooking* style, with the ingredients listed in bold so you can make your shopping list easily, some recipes just called for being written in story form. And some have just the ingredients listed without any amounts, to get you thinking! Or using what you have.

At the beginning of each season you will find a list of recipes included in that section, in alphabetical order. At the back of the book you will find an alphabetical list for *all* the recipes and menus in the book. In the back you will also find a list of all recipes in groupings. These aren't the common ones, like appetizers or main dishes, because I have found that since vegetarian cooking is not centered around meat, it has much more flow.

I have grouped things both by content (**Pasta, Potatoes, and Rice**, all high starch foods), cooking method (**Chilies, Curries, and Stews**, all similar except for the spices and ingredients), or special function (**Toppings, Sauces, Gravy, and Stuffing**, all things Marlo Morgan's *Real People* would laugh at as superfluous).

Volume Cooking and Preserving is a separate category, though many of the recipes in this book are for amounts large enough to freeze for later (or for a large family). Many of the recipes in this book are based on using frozen basic ingredients, such as rice, tomatoes, broth, or beans, so try your hand at all of these. If you come to a recipe and you don't have items already in the freezer, you can look ahead to next year. In the meantime, substitute commercially prepared items, such as frozen vegetables, or occasionally canned.

All the little tidbits of food prep or nutrition that I've learned from cooks or doctors along the way are listed in the grouping **X-tras** for easy reference, though much of my cooking experience comes out in the recipes themselves.

Following this note is a lengthy explanation of various oddities about the cookbook that others who read early drafts were confused by. Most of these are personal idiosyncrasies, but don't we all have those? If you're a blank slate, take on some of mine if you want to. But if you're already an experienced cook, substitute your own for mine as you read and cook. Be my guest! And be in touch. Sally@SallyMiller.com.

Abbreviations, Substitutions, and Equivalents

evoo = extra virgin olive oil
t = teaspoon
T = tablespoon
C = cup
pt = pint
qt = quart

Substitute This   **for This**

frozen cranberries   fresh cranberries
frozen blueberries   fresh blueberries
frozen raspberries   fresh raspberries
green beans chopped small   fresh or frozen peas
hemp, soy or rice milk   almond milk

1 T = 3 t	16 oz = 1 lb
2 T = 1/8 C (coffee scoop)	1/4 lb = 1 stick butter
4 T = 1/4 C	4 oz = 1 stick
8 T = 1/2 C	4 oz = 1/2 C butter
16 T = 1 C	2 C = 1 pint (pt)
48 t = 1 C = 16 T	2 pts = 1 quart (qt)

3 ears corn ≈ 2 C corn   4 ears corn ≈ 2 2/3 C corn
3 handfuls pasta ≈ 1 C (measure your own & adjust accordingly)
1 T fresh herb   ≈ 1 t dried herb
1 C raw vegetable   ≈ 1/2 C cooked (serving size)
1/2 C applesauce or 1 small banana ≈ 1/2 C fat in baking recipe
1 T lime juice   ≈ 1 lime squeezed
3/4 C whole wheat flour ≈ 1 C white flour

dice means to cut into strips, then into small cubes ≈ 1/4"
mince means to dice really small; *finely minced* is smaller still
chop means to cut into smaller than bite-size pieces; coarser than dice, not as precise
flake means to break up into small bits with a fork

Pecans and Limes
A Note of Explanation

Why do I use pecans and cashews instead of other kinds of nuts, like walnuts (whose shells make the greatest little boats) or almonds? The answer is simple — my teeth. Almonds and walnuts are both more nutritious, with less fat. But if your teeth are precarious like mine, you stick to something softer. Anyway, pecans go back a long way in my family. Use whatever nuts you like and have on hand when you meet a nut in a recipe.

As for limes, I much prefer them to lemons. I'll never forget one of the first times my husband Roger went shopping for our family of six, and Pledge the dust sprayer was on the list. He brought home Lemon Pledge — and I've been off lemons ever since. Whether it was the artificial smell I didn't like but always associated with real lemons, or something from my childhood, who knows? I just didn't like it. I used ReaLemon when a recipe called for lemon juice, and just left out any zest asked for. But I tended to avoid it altogether as much as I could.

It wasn't until fairly recently that I started using limes — perhaps because Hispanic culture has finally moved into New Jersey. We are seeing an influx of food from Latino cultures such as Mexican, Costa Rican, Puerto Rican, Jamaican, and Cuban, to name a few. Each has its distinct foods, but many of them use similar ingredients which lime juice has a natural affinity towards. Suddenly limes and tortillas are everywhere. Viva Latinos! Except here we call tortillas *wraps*.

Some other unusual choices for me: almond and hempseed milk as non-dairy liquids, and canned coconut milk. All are easily stored in my big cupboard with few canned/processed foods. I like the look and taste of almond milk much better than soy, which is often used as a milk substitute. We don't want to use milk because cow's milk was made for baby cows. It also encourages breast, ovarian, testicular, and prostate cancers. Coconut milk is high fat, but I use the thick top for desserts and the low-fat part for curries.

A food I mention over and over is little red potatoes, which I especially like. They are more nutritious than large brown potatoes because of their higher ratio of skin to potato meat: skin is real natural fiber and there are more nutrients near the skin. This is even more so if the brown potatoes are peeled (try mashed potatoes leaving the skin on): peeling potatoes removes all that fiber and nutrition. Feel free to substitute as you wish.

Another item I use profusely is the Vidalia onion. I first found out about Vidalia onions from young chef Brian who worked for me several years. As usual, I was not very experimental with food, but at his suggestion I tried them. Their season is in the spring and summer, and they are grown only around Vidalia, Georgia. They are milder than my old stand-by, yellow onions, and Vidalia onions are perfect for salads. In the winter try sweet onions from Peru.

I almost always say "yams" and not "sweet potatoes." There is much debate over the differences between yams and sweet potatoes. What you should use is the darkest meat of sweet potatoes/yams you can find. Buy one of each at your produce market and cut them all open to see. At mine the darkest orange "potatoes" have the darkest skin. My Korean green grocer Neil calls them *yams*, so I do, also. The darker the color, the more nutrients there are.

Dressing and *stuffing*. Aha! Growing up my older sister would call it "stuffing," and our mother would correct her to "dressing." I believe dressing was considered more refined (and therefore more worthy of our usage of it), but nowadays, I don't think it matters that much. I treat them interchangeably. Answers.com says the following: "After about 1880, the term *stuffing* was replaced by *dressing* in Victorian English. Both terms are used today." Since our mother prided herself in properness, I can now see why she preferred *dressing*.

I use organic potato flakes to thicken instead of flour. I use Sucanat (**Sugar Cane Natural**) instead of white sugar (you'll have to ask a vegan for the reasons for this one). I also use Grade B maple syrup for a sweetener in cooking because it is richer in nutrients than Grade A, though Grade A is sweeter and better for pancakes.

I choose low sodium tamari sauce over regular soy sauce for health reasons, a vegetable brush (which I wash in the dishwasher every so often) over a sponge after watching a 20/20 program years ago about sponges smearing filth around the kitchen. I use paper towels to wipe my cutting boards and my counters. *Frequently.* Perhaps someday paper towels will be made out of industrial hemp, an easily renewable green resource, rather than trees, which are not.

Evoo means *extra virgin olive oil*. This and *smashing the garlic* are terms I got from Rachel Ray, whose first year of "30-Minute Meals" cooking program on The Food Channel was such an inspiration to me. At that time Rachel was less talk-show host and more high vegetarian Mediterranean-diet chef, who talked fast and giggled, as I have been accused of doing over the years. I smash my garlic with a power stone which I also use for sharpening knives. Smashing allows for speedy removal of the skin from a clove of garlic, particularly if you cut the end off first before you smash. The clove can then be sliced or diced easily, and the essence of the garlic is more accessible.

Substitute Swiss chard for kale if it looks better — fresher — than the kale. Vice versa. If Vidalia onions aren't available, use shallots or yellow or purple onion (use less of these last two). After a while you'll get so you can tell what is freshest. Ask your produce person where the fruit or vegetable comes from. That tells you alot, but I wouldn't rule out something from South America. Their growing season is just the opposite of ours, and with free trade, produce moves more quickly. But I will admit I always like it when I spy the first Florida blueberries!

I talk some about puff pastry. In my twenties I watched Julia Child making it on TV (now on YouTube). I tried it, but it sure was work! Now Pepperidge Farm puts out a puff pastry made with canola oil. Though not as good as the butter kind, it is certainly less work! And vegan. I can also get real puff pastry in bulk at Thai restaurants where they have Curry Puffs on the menu.

As to freezer containers, I am completely sold on using the plastic soup containers I can get from my favorite Chinese restaurant. Substitute whatever you want, but make sure you never heat your food in them (thawing is okay).

What on earth does "picked over" mean? Well, you wash the berries or beans well in a colander under running water, then go through them, tossing out any scrunched up, shriveled, funny-colored berry or bean and picking off any stems left on. Wash again, shaking the colander to uncover any less than perfect berry/bean.

Speaking of washing, I emphasize scrubbing carrots and potatoes (with a brush) while rarely mentioning other vegetables, because potatoes and carrots are the vegetables most likely to be peeled by mainstream cooks to the depreciation of nutrition. Please remember, however, that even though I don't mention it in every recipe, ALL fruits and vegetables should be washed before using.

The best kitchen invention of recent times is the immersion blender. As with many other things, I learned about this from Brian, a chef in another life. A functional one from Braun (like the white one hanging up on the cover of this book) runs around $20, and you can order just the cutting blade section for $6 (it does get dull). A more elaborate one (Smart Stick) made by Cuisinart runs $35, and it comes with a chopper attachment. It is well worth the difference in price for the chopper, but it *is* heavier and more difficult to use.

I use virtually no salt because it is healthier, though tamari sauce provides saltiness for various dishes. There are a few foods that seem to need salt, however, like potatoes and some soups, and I usually mention this in a recipe. Try to keep your salt usage to a minimum, as it can be toxic to the system (I know a gravely ill woman who speeded her death with salt water).

Finally, you may find me using the words "outloud" and "alot." I think both of these should be one word, no matter what the dictionary and grammar book say. So I've used them that way.

If there's anything else you don't understand or want to know more about, look on the web or send me an email at Sally@SallyMiller.com.

Sally's
in the
Kitchen

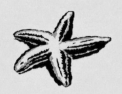

SUMMER

June, July, August

Summer

Much of my extra activity in the kitchen beyond meal preparations comes mid to late summer, when the local farmers are producing tomatoes and corn and squash, as well as blueberries from South Jersey, all wonderful for stocking the freezer. I work in front of the air conditioner, and most days have help. Summer's the time to freeze garden bounty.

If you don't have a freezer, get one. My first freezer was a small chest freezer. I lived in an apartment, and got it secondhand for $75. I used the top of it for projects I wanted to lay out and look at. Eventually it gave out and I got an upright freezer for free from someone who didn't want to take it cross country in its banged-up but working condition. It still works fine. I could use a second one, actually, as I have no freezer space in my "vegetarian reefer" — a refrigerator that has no freezer on top, bottom, or side. Just cold, with four crispers!

I keep one freezer shelf for broth, tomato sauce, rice, beans, and other ready-to-use items. One shelf is for ready-made, warm-only soups, stews, chilis, curries, casseroles, etc. I keep things I don't [want to] eat that often, such as butter, shredded cheese, ground meat, bread, and cookies, frozen on a bottom shelf.

I actually got my first separate freezer when I cooked for a family of six. In it I kept a beef quarter, pork cuts, and raw/cooked chicken ready to prepare. I cooked ahead for a rainy day, and I had prepared meals for a month when my youngest child was born and first home. Later that same freezer became home to stacks and stacks of Stouffers during my "Sex and the Suburbs" days. Then I moved several times and didn't think I had the room for a freezer, changing my ways of cooking and thinking ahead, of preserving for bad weather days. Boy, am I glad I got back to storing fresh and freshly cooked foods in the freezer! For a working gal the benefits are huge. I can cook large pots of something, freeze in pint containers, and later simply warm something over the stove in a small saucepan while the rice is defrosting and I am answering my email!

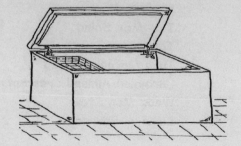

Hinky Dink

A sandwich spread that always signified the start of summer and warm weather to me growing up in Iowa — the start of wearing white and swimsuits, of having no school. This old family recipe was traditionally made and served for Memorial Day picnics, but in our family it was also served at VEISHEA, the Iowa State student extravaganza held in May each year.

Because my birthday is in May, too, I also associate hinky dink with the beginning of a new year (and now, the start of a new cookbook). I have been unable to find anyone else who has this recipe, except perhaps the numerous student girls who worked for room and board at our house while I was growing up.

Original recipe, with no directions:

- 1/4 lb (4 oz) cheddar cheese
- 3 sweet pickles
- 1/2 C peanuts
- 1 pimento
- 1/2 lemon
- Miracle whip to spread

I always make at least 4 x the original recipe:
- 1 lb cheddar cheese
- 12 sweet pickles
- 2 C peanuts
- 4 pimentos (2 4-oz jars)

Put these four ingredients through a hand grinder, with a bowl below (on the floor or on a stool) to catch drips. Use a medium or large blade, so there are some little chunks (as in chunky peanut butter). Run some dried heels of bread or crackers through at the end to clean out the grinder. Add:
- **2 lemons,** juice and zest
- **Miracle Whip** (mayonnaise if you must) to moisten

Will firm up in refrigerator, and more Miracle Whip may need to be added when serving. Use on crackers, in sandwiches (especially on rye bread), on little hors d'oeuvre-size bread, Rye Crisp, bagel chips, or Nooni.

Orange Mint Drink

An old family recipe, revised. Makes a concentrate that can be used when unexpected company arrives during the late spring or summer after the mint has come up. I fondly call this a Shirley Temple mint julep.

Make a sugar syrup from:
> **3 C water**
> **1 1/2 C Sucanat**

Cook and stir over medium heat until it comes to a boil.

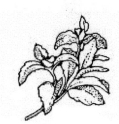

Meanwhile, strip from stem and wash:
> **2 handfuls of mint leaves**

Place in a large metal, glass, or hard pottery bowl. Scrub well with a brush:
> **2 oranges**
> **2 lemons**
> **1 lime**

Using a fine grater, grate rind of fruits into bowl (zest). Cut each fruit in half and juice with a hand juicer into bowl. Then cut each carcass into 4 pieces and add to bowl. Pour hot sugar syrup over fruit-and-mint mixture in bowl.

Let sit for 20 - 30 minutes. Longer than this and it may become bitter. Add:
> **2 cups fresh orange juice**

Strain into 2-quart covered pitcher or large jar with cover.

When ready to serve, put sprig of fresh mint into a tall glass. Fill with ice cubes. Pour glass one half full with concentrate. Fill with plain water, tonic water, or carbonated water. Add drink stirrer or straw and garnish with a fresh sprig of mint. This is a drink to be nursed, a sipping drink.

Leave room for a shot of bourbon if you want a more authentic julep taste. Or try gin or tequila. Store leftovers of concentrate in refrigerator up to 2 weeks.

No mint patch? Buy one of the many varieties available or get some from a friend. It will spread readily wherever you plant it, so you need to keep it in check or it will take over an herb garden. My mint was originally a gift from my sister Martha (from North Dakota), who got it from our mother's mint (in Iowa), which came from her mother's (in Oklahoma) which came from HER mother's (in Kansas). Who knows before that? I have carried a new starting of it wherever I have moved.

Fruit Drink

For each drink use **1 ripe banana**, some kind of **berry** (about 1/2 a cup), and **one other fruit**.

Peel banana and break into 4 or 5 pieces. Set aside for ease in adding later. Put berries such as strawberries, blueberries, or grapes into pitcher or other suitable container. Cut up and add other fruit, preferably with skin on if the skin is thin (like peach, apple, kiwi). Barely cover with orange juice or other fruit juice. Blend with an immersion blender until smooth. Add banana pieces and blend again. Pour and drink. Super good, and nutritious. I "eat" this for breakfast nearly every morning, supplemented with toast & almond butter if I'm still hungry.

During high allergy season or during the winter when house is closed up with pets, use 1 clementine, 1 slice or 4 big chunks fresh pineapple, blueberries, 1 banana, orange juice or pineapple juice.

The clementine and pineapple both supply *quercetin*, which is a natural anti-histamine that stops the formation of histamine on a cellular level (rather than treating the symptoms after they have appeared with a drying, habit-forming, toxic pharmaceutical).

People with allergies generally have too acidic a system, and would do well to increase both raw vegetables and raw fruits.

I serve this drink to my assistants, who often come to work without eating breakfast. (Actually, they make it and serve it to me!)

This along with **Garden Salad** (page 21) are two of the most important recipes in this book. Add a daily fruit drink and a garden salad to your diet and you will change your acidity to a healthier number; all your illnesses will lessen, your wellness will increase.

Mediterranean Potato Salad

My vegan friend Arnie first fixed this for me out of the vegan cookbook from Veggie Works, our favorite restaurant down the shore in Belmar NJ. I adapted it and often serve it with a large green salad that has cut-up vegetables (such as cucumbers, tomatoes, broccoli, cauliflower, and radishes) on top of the salad greens. Though I always put out small bowls for guests to put the potato salad in, they usually end up spooning this delicious potato salad on top as a "dressing" to the green/vegetable salad.

Scrub and trim (but don't peel):

12 medium red potatoes (20 small)

Cook in water to cover until almost tender. Drain off water and save in freezer for soup. When potatoes are cool enough to handle, cube (or quarter if small) and place in large bowl. Add:

1/2 red onion, chopped

1 rib celery, minced

1 green bell pepper, diced

1 C fresh peas

1 carrot, shredded

Top with:

4 T extra virgin olive oil (evoo) or other fine oil

3 T apple cider vinegar

1 t salt

1/2 t black pepper

Mix well, chill, mix again, and serve. Keeps well.

Pasta Salad

The only pasta I ever ate growing up was Kraft Dinner with elbow macaroni, and once a year my mother's "Italian spaghetti," with the long spaghetti noodles everyone is familiar with. After I moved to New Jersey, especially in Hunterdon County, I discovered dozens of other kinds of pasta. With a large Italian immigrant population and their descendents, even the local grocery stores supply dozens of shapes, ingredients and brands to choose from. For a while we even had a Sopranos-type Italian specialty store where you could almost smell Italy inside. What wonderful fresh pasta and vegetables!

Nowadays I keep six or seven pastas on hand to suit my mood. If I want something substantial, I choose Campanelle; if I want something light, I use mixed vermicelli. I can also choose vegetable twists, mixed white and whole wheat bows, fusilli, wheat shells from Italy, or some other kind of pasta.

Cook until tender:

5 handfuls pasta ($\approx$ 2 C)

Drain well in a colander. Place in serving bowl.

Shred and add:

1 carrot

1 onion

Dice and add:

2 Kirby cucumbers (small, or pickling cukes)

2 dill pickles

2 ribs celery

1 medium green zucchini

Mix gently. Add:

Miracle Whip or mayonnaise to moisten.

Decorate top of salad with:

hard-cooked egg, sliced

When I was trying to learn to like zucchini raw, I started adding it to this version of an old family potato salad recipe.

Picnic Bean Salad

A woman I met through a day retreat at Boxelder Basin Wellness Center brought me a 25-lb box of dried pinto beans as a gift. I often cooked enough at one time to freeze many pints of beans and juice, which I used for months and months instead of canned beans. Better tasting, and better for you! If you've cooked and frozen beans throughout the year, just grab a couple of containers from your freezer.

This is a salad that my mother made with canned dark red kidney beans. In the summer we'd pack a picnic basket and head to the Ledges, a state park not that far from where we lived. Here we could hike and dip our feet in the cold creek that ran throughout the park, including over some of the winding park road. What fun it was to drive through the water, usually no more than an inch or two, and watch it splash up.

Use **2 pints (4 cups) of cooked pinto or kidney beans.** Drain, rinse, and place in large mixing bowl. Dice and add:

> **4 dill pickles**
> **4 Kirby cucumbers** (the little short ones) *
> **2 hard-boiled eggs** (vegans can leave out)
> **1 small green zucchini** *
> **1 small yellow zucchini** *
> **1/2 stalk celery** (cut across ribs, leaves and all)
> **1/2 head cauliflower** *
> **1 onion or 6 - 8 scallions**

Add:

> **2 shredded carrots** *

Mix well. Add dressing (**mayonnaise or Miracle Whip**), mixing well. Chill. Enjoy.

* Things I added to my mother's bean salad to make it more nutritious.

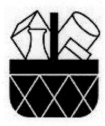

Fourth of July Baked Beans

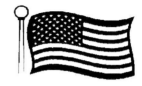

Cook at night when the air conditioning is off.

Place the following in a large soup pot:

    12 C mixed cooked beans (kidney, pinto, Great Northern, black) ≈ 2 lbs dry
    carrots, onions & celery, approximately 2 cups each
    1 C split peas
    1 C dark molasses (blackstrap)
    1/4 C tomato sauce
    1/4 C honey or maple syrup
    4 t mustard

Add vegetable broth and/or water to cover beans. Heat on stovetop, stirring well, then place in a 300° oven for 4 - 6 hours, stirring occasionally. Add water and adjust seasoning if needed.

Take to Fourth of July picnic in a large bean pot or crockpot. Freeze rest for the winter doldrums.

Pico de Gallo
"Peeko day guy-o"

Brian, one of my young assistants, first showed me how to make pico de gallo. When tomatoes come into season it is one of my favorite foods, and I eat it often. A big batch can age in the refrigerator and be available at any time. Keep a big bag of restaurant-style Tostido chips in your cupboard with a chip clip to keep them fresh. Then when you don't feel like cooking but you're hungry, grab a chip and scoop yourself up some vitamin C.

    4 plum tomatoes, small dice
    1 cucumber, small dice
    1 jalapeño pepper, finely minced
    a little onion and garlic
    fresh cilantro
    salt and pepper
    juice of one lime

Mix together and let chill. Serve with chips, preferably ones baked, not fried.

Paul's Chicken

If your body is craving chicken, get chicken from your local Amish community or farmers market. Have them skin and cut into pieces — each breast cut in half, then in half again, so each piece is small. Include legs, thighs, and wings cut apart (discard wing tips). I devised this recipe years ago when my son Paul, the youngest of four children, was little. He loved it, as did the rest of the family. Now I usually have it on July 23, his birthday, and perhaps again in the winter.

Preheat oven to 350°

Wash, dry and skin:
> **organic chicken parts**

Shake in gallon-size Ziploc bag a few pieces at a time with equal parts of:
> **bread crumbs**
> **parmesan cheese**

Place chicken pieces in baking dish. Drizzle with equal parts of:
> **melted butter**
> **olive oil**

Put in preheated oven for 20 minutes.

Turn chicken pieces with tongs.

Bake another 10 - 15 minutes or until lightly browned and crispy.

Serve with egg noodles (make plenty to soak up all the crumbs and butter) and a green vegetable like peas or broccoli.

Freeze leftovers in meal-size containers to have when you crave chicken, or to have available for a guest who "needs" meat.

Perfect Veggie Burger

When I was growing up we had hamburgers almost every Saturday night (occasionally we had Mexican Buns instead). This is my modern-day version of the Saturday night burger, a healthy version you can serve any day of the week.

1 wheat potato or buckwheat hamburger roll (sliced in half)
dressing of your choice (ketchup, mustard, mayo, or my favorite,
      Miracle Whip)
pickle slices
1 slice tomato
spinach leaves (washed well)
1 slice raw onion
1 portobello mushroom (de-stemmed and sautéed in evoo)
2 leaves of leafy lettuce (remove rib if hard)

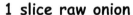

If you don't like raw onion, sauté onion with the mushroom.

Start with bottom of bun, pickle slices, tomato, spinach, and onion. Then add your mushroom "hamburger" and put curly lettuce leaves on top. Cap with toasted bun top.

Mexican Buns

Brown **1 pound ground chuck,** chopping meat up into small pieces. Drain fat from pan. Add **1/2 C piccalilli** (sweet pickle relish) and **1/2 C chili sauce** (salsa). Stir and simmer for ten minutes. Add **1/2 C grated cheddar cheese.** When cheese has melted, spoon into buns and eat with gusto! Makes enough filling for six hamburger buns.

Tex-Mex Bean Salad

Yummy summer salad. If you have frozen corn and dried mint, it's good anytime.

> 4 C cooked beans (roman, pinto, black, Great Northern, etc.)
> 4 ears corn, cooked & stripped (2 1/2 - 3 C)
> 1 green pepper, small diced
> 1 red pepper, small diced
> 1 handful fresh mint, stripped and chopped
> 1 t cumin
> 1/2 t ground coriander
> juice of 2 lemons
> 1/3 C olive oil

Mix all ingredients together and chill.

Quick Salads

For each person, shred:
> 1 carrot, scrubbed and ends trimmed
> 1 small cucumber (Kirby), scrubbed and ends trimmed
> 1 small onion, peeled

QS 2: 1 large carrot
> 2 radishes
> 1/2 Kirby cucumber

Add:
> 1 - 2 t dressing

Toss, chill, and serve.

I use Miracle Whip for this recipe, but you can use any kind of dressing you wish, including oil and vinegar, soy mayonnaise, etc.

QS 3: 1/4 head romaine lettuce
> 1 Kirby cuke
> 1 carrot
> 1/2 onion

Top with dressing or a dollop of leftover bean salad, potato or pasta salad, or any of the chilis listed in the index by grouping.

Stuffed Mushrooms

Once in a while I feel like having something elegant. This is it. I found the original recipe in our local newspaper, The Observer.

Preheat oven to 375°

Clean with a brush, pat dry, and remove stems (save) from:
> **8 large white mushrooms**

Use of a curved grapefruit knife makes this easier. After loosening stem, grab hold with your fingers and wiggle it out, removing enough to make a nice cavity for filling. Place mushrooms in an oval baking dish, stem side up.

In a blender grind:
> **saved mushroom stems**
> **2 cloves garlic,** peeled
> **1/2 slice whole grain bread,** dried and broken into pieces
> **6 walnuts or almonds**

Add and process until well combined:
> **2 T rosemary**
> **2 T parsley**
> **2 T extra virgin olive oil (evoo)**

Season to taste with salt and pepper if desired.

Divide filling between the 8 caps. Bake for 20 - 25 minutes or until golden brown.

Tuna Macaroni Salad

> **1 12-oz box macaroni**
> **1/2 onion,** finely minced
> **1/2 stalk of celery,** washed & cut across stalk (leaves and all)
> **1 large carrot,** grated
> **10 Spanish green olives with pimento,** sliced
> **1 7-oz can tuna,** drained

Cook macaroni. Drain. Add other ingredients and mayo or Miracle Whip to moisten. Mix well and chill.

Bruschetta

The American pronunciation is *broo-SHEH-tah;* in Italian it's this wonderful guttural *broo-SCHKEH-tah.*

I was introduced to bruschetta the summer I had my first-year celebration of life after surviving ovarian cancer. While traveling north through New York State and Canada in late August, I found bruschetta on the menu everywhere I went. My favorite version, served as a hearty hors d'oeuvre, was from the Carriage House Restaurant in downtown Watertown, New York.

Now every July when the tomatoes and peppers first come out, this is one of my favorite foods (I've taken liberties with their recipe). I have it for a whole meal, savoring the various flavors and temperatures.

Wash, trim, core, and dice into small pieces (but do not skin):
>   **6 beautiful firm red tomatoes** (or 12 plum tomatoes)

Place in a medium-size bowl. Wash, dice, and add to bowl:
>   **1 large firm green pepper**

Add and mix in:
>   **1/2 C organic extra-virgin olive oil** (evoo)
>   **1/2 C bottled Wishbone Italian salad dressing**
>   **2 T fresh basil,** chopped (or 1 - 2 t dried & crumbled)
>   **1 T fresh oregano,** chopped (or 1 t dried & crumbled)
>   **2 cloves garlic,** finely minced or pressed

Refrigerate for at least 4 hours, or overnight, stirring occasionally.

When ready to serve, preheat broiler. Slice lengthwise:
>   **1 long skinny loaf whole grain bread**

Cut each half in two and place cut side down on broiler-friendly baking pan or heavy CorningWare. Toast the outside of loaf until crusty brown, especially important if loaf is soft to the touch. Turn bread over and lightly toast on top. Remove from broiler. (Both this step and the tomato step can be done ahead of time, making this an ideal dish for company.)

To assemble, cut each toasted piece of bread in half. Place a top and matching bottom piece in shallow broiler-proof bowl or plate, cut sides up. (Each serving will therefore be 1/4 of the original loaf.)

Spoon liberal amounts of tomato mixture onto both pieces in each bowl. Top with:
shelled hempseeds (Nutiva brand available at most health food stores)

You can also use a small amount of grated parmesan cheese or jalepeño soy cheese. Pop into the broiler for a minute or two, until seeds brown slightly or cheese melts. Serve immediately with a knife and fork. Serves 4.

I have substituted a freshly diced onion for the green pepper at times, or used a small cucumber or zucchini squash, diced fine. In a pinch I've used thick slices of bread, toasted, but it always seems like a poor cousin to the real thing. Leftover juices and bits can be used to dress a green salad.

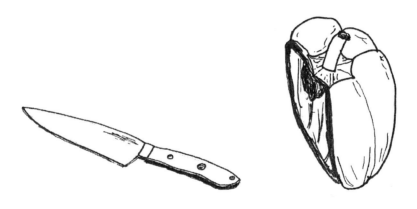

Hold pepper straight up and down, with stem end up. Slice as large a slice as you can from one side, cutting from top to bottom, curving your cut slightly with the curve of the pepper. Push slice aside and turn pepper, making another slice from top to bottom. Continue to turn and slice until all you have left is the core, which you can nibble on before you toss it into the compost. Cut each slice into strips, then cut across the strips to make little squares (dice). Once you learn how to dice a pepper this way, you'll never do it the messy, old-fashioned way again!

Cucumbers and Cream

This is used as a topping for boiled potatoes, a favorite summer dish from my childhood. My father used to slice and salt the cukes in the morning before he went to work, then when he came home for lunch he would squeeze them out. After lunch my mother would make the sauce and let everything chill till dinnertime. Served with pork chops (p.104) in the past, but I like to serve with a black bean salad (p.121).

Scrub, trim ends, and score lengthwise with a fork:

4 fresh cucumbers

With a sharp paring knife slice each cucumber very thin into a flat bowl, sprinkling liberally with salt as you go along. Let sit on the counter for 3 - 4 hours, turning cucumbers over occasionally. Water will magically appear! When water is ample and cucumbers are soft, take the cucumbers, a small handful at a time, and squeeze the water out (into the sink is fine), putting squeezed ones into a second bowl. Squeeze them all again, one handful at a time, placing back into first bowl. Rinse out second bowl and add:

1 to 1 1/2 C cream (amount depending on size of cucumbers)

1 T to 2 T vinegar

Stir until cream looks thick (almost like commercial sour cream). Add cucumbers, squeezing again before adding. Mix well, and chill for 2 - 4 hours in refrigerator. Season as desired. Sometimes I add fresh mint, chopped.

There's no getting around it, you can't make good cucumbers and cream without using cream. Real cream. We used to use "top milk," or the cream that rose to the top of the milk bottle before homogenization. Half and half will suffice, but medium or heavy cream is better. Watch your fat calories for the rest of the week if you make this recipe!

Quick Pix

Use **fat short cucumbers** for this wonderful salad. Score the skins with a fork and trim the ends. Cut lengthwise into quarters, remove majority of seeds, cut each spear in half, then into chunks. Cover with mixture of **half rice vinegar, half water, with a little maple syrup** to take the edge off the vinegar. You can add any kind of **herb** you like, though I make mine plain. Keep in the refrigerator for 3 - 4 hours or longer. Eat as is, or put on top of salad greens. Yummy!

Hot Cucumber Salad
(spicy hot that is)

For that hot day!

1 C colored peppers, minced
2 cucumbers, chopped
1 plum tomato, chopped
1 small onion, chopped
1 jalapeño pepper, finely minced

Mix and add a little evoo and vinegar.

Dill Pickles

This came from a friend who also has a garden and looks for ways to use her bountiful produce in the summer. Thanks, Patty!

Do you have fresh dill? Buy some if you don't have it. Make pickles! Very simple recipe.

Wash and dry 4 pint-size jars and tops in the dishwasher to sterilize them. Wash the cucumbers and pack them into the hot jars. You can cut them to fit if needed or just use them chunked up or whole if they are small. For one jar slice the cucumbers to use on burgers.

Place **a fresh dill sprig and a clove of garlic** in each jar. Use **6 cups water, 2 cups white vinegar, 1/2 cup salt** (table or coarse) for four pints pickles. Boil the water, vinegar and salt in a *non-aluminum pan*, pour over the cucumbers and seal. Put away in a cool place for 6 weeks (mark your calendar!) and you can chill and eat. No other processing required.

I found the only problem was waiting that 6 weeks to eat them!

Patty adds: I also tried adding chunky cukes to minestrone for the last few minutes of cooking the soup . . . it was a great addition.

5-Year Celebration of Life
Menu
August 12, 2001

*All items vegan except as noted *

Beans & Swiss Chard Stew (opposite page)
Irish Potato Bake (p.97)
Bow-Tie Pasta Salad * (p.5)
Orange Mint Drink (p.2)
Lemon Lime Drink
Almond-Butter Cookies (p.48)
Arnie's Rice Dish
Garden Salad (p.21)

Beans & Swiss Chard Stew

Soak overnight:

 2 C dried pinto beans, washed & picked over

In morning rinse well and put in large soup pot with water to cover by 2".
Add:

 1/2 C dried green split peas, washed & picked over

Bring to a boil, turn down heat, and simmer for an hour.
Add:

 1/2 stalk celery, washed & cut across all ribs, leaves & all

 4 carrots, scrubbed, trimmed & cut into rounds

 1 large onion, diced

Stir and add water as necessary, cooking until beans are tender.
Add:

 6 - 10 large green Swiss chard, washed, trimmed & cut across leaves and stems.

 6 - 10 radishes, washed & cut into thin rounds

 6 - 10 small potatoes, scrubbed & sliced

Cook until it reaches a consistency you like. I usually cook until potatoes are fork tender. Remove from heat and let cool. It will thicken more upon sitting. For thicker beans, cook until split pea hulls are broken down and sauce is smooth, adding chard, radishes, and small potatoes later. Spice as desired or serve plain.

I served this at my 5th annual Celebration of Life Open House. Then I neglected chard for years till my wood man brought it back into my life.

Summer Buffet

Zucchini Rounds (p.18)
Boiled Little Red Potatoes
Cucumbers & Cream w/Mint (p.14)
Berry Cherry Bowl w/Coconut Cream (p.112)

Zucchini Rounds

This is my favorite recipe when zucchini hits the garden with a bang! I can eat this every day.

Preheat oven to 350°

Mix **1 cup bread crumbs** with **1 cup grated parmesan cheese.** (Parmigiano-Reggiano makes it even better.)

Lightly coat the bottom of a 9" x 13" baking pan with **olive oil**.

Wash **large zucchini squash** well, trimming off ends (a smaller squash will need a smaller pan). Cut rounds of squash about 1/2" thick (do not peel). Squash cut thicker will come out a bit firmer; thinner rounds may become too mushy. Place rounds in prepared baking pan so that entire bottom is covered with rounds. Turn each round over so that both tops and bottoms have a very thin coating of olive oil.

Sprinkle crumb mixture on top of rounds. Any remaining crumb mixture can be refrigerated for future use.

Bake in 350° oven for 30 minutes.

Serve and enjoy.

Can be baked in CorningWare or other flat casserole dish if you will be serving at the table. Kids and guests love to help with this.

Crumbs

Make crumbs out of dried whole-grain bread, stale corn chips, bagel chips, crackers, tortilla chips, or whatever you have in your kitchen. I usually use an old blender I keep for just this purpose (I leave heels of bread here to dry out), or you can put chips and hunks of dried bread into a large heavy plastic bag that zips closed and roll with a rolling pin or pound with a wooden mallet.

Tomatoes

To make a delicious tomato sauce, use any kind of really ripe tomato — heirloom, Rutgers, cherry, Italian or plum, beefsteak, or any ordinary garden variety of tomato. I usually do a bushel at a time, getting them from my more productive neighbors, though I often add tomatoes from my garden.

In a Dutch oven over low heat cook cored and trimmed tomatoes cut into half or large chunks (leave skin on). Keep adding tomatoes until tomatoes come nearly to the top of the pan. Cook over low heat until cooked down and saucy, adding more tomatoes as you go along. Stir frequently until tomatoes are soft and incorporated with the liquid they've produced (or ladle off "water" and save in freezer for soups).

Blend to incorporate the seeds and skins, as this is where the most nutrition lies. If you want a chunky sauce, pulse your blender. Blend longer for a smoother sauce. If sauce is too thin, cook over low heat until thicker. Use as is or freeze in pint-size Chinese soup containers for future use. Can be used in soups, pizza sauce, and vegetable pasta sauces. Freeze some sauce in an ice-cube tray (transfer to plastic bag or container when frozen) to use when you need only a tablespoon or two of sauce.

For a pizza sauce, add onion, garlic, pepper, oregano, and basil. Recipe page 143.

$20.00 worth of fresh organic field grown tomatoes = 14 pints of sauce in 2008.
$15.00 worth of fresh organic field grown tomatoes = 11 pints of sauce in 2008.

Average cost of sauce/pint (without electricity, container or time) $1.40

I have a good friend who freezes her tomato bounty raw, in chunks and whole, for processing later. I prefer to do the cooking at one time (once or twice a week during tomato season I cook a large pot of tomatoes and freeze containers of tomatoes for the winter and spring).

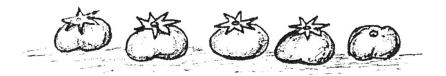

Ukrainian Almond Crescents

I made these for a Ukrainian author I was working with who came to visit with his family. Unfortunately his mother, who at 85 still spoke fluent Ukrainian, had gall bladder problems and was unable to eat them. But they were/are delicious!

2 – 2 1/2 cups flour, unbleached or whole wheat
1 package dry yeast
1 cup sweet butter, room temperature
2 egg yolks, beaten (save whites)
1/4 cup sour cream

For the pastry, mix together the flour and yeast in a medium bowl. Cut in the butter with a pastry fork until the mixture resembles coarse meal. Stir in the egg yolks and sour cream and mix well. The mixture will still be crumbly. Form the dough into a ball using your hands, working it as little as possible. The less you knead, the more tender the pastry will be. The dough will be tacky. Wrap it in waxed paper and chill it for at least 2 hours.

Filling:
2 cups almonds, toasted and coarsely ground
2/3 cup brown sugar, firmly packed (3/4 C Sucanat)
2 egg whites
1 pinch salt

Prepare the filling by combining the ground almonds and sugar in a small bowl. Beat together the egg whites and salt in a medium bowl until stiff, but not dry, and carefully fold the nut mixture into them.

When the dough has thoroughly chilled, preheat oven to 350° and divide the dough into three balls. Using a floured rolling pin, roll out three circles about 1/8" thick. Work on a well-floured surface to prevent the dough from sticking. Spread 1/3 of the filling on each circle. Cut each circle into eight pie-shaped wedges, and starting at the wide end, roll each wedge up like a horn and then pull the ends into a curve to form a crescent. Make sure the point is on the bottom so the "horns" will not open up while baking. Place the almond crescents on a lightly oiled baking sheet and bake for about 20 to 25 minutes, until golden and puffed. Makes 24

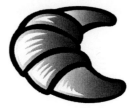

As my friend Brice would say, a coronary made in heaven!

Garden Salad

I have discovered the secret to having garden salad ready to eat any time without sacrificing quality. It utilizes the antibiotic characteristics of raw onion, and made according to my directions, will keep a week in the refrigerator (if you make enough, that is!). I try to eat a salad every day.

Get the freshest greens possible. I always start with a base of leafy lettuce: one week I get the dark reddish kind, the next week I get the green leafy kind, and the third week I get Romaine. All of these have superior nutrition to iceberg lettuce, which is the least nutrient-dense lettuce there is. Lettuce is washed and broken into pieces small enough for me to get into my mouth without seeming like a caveman. I place all of these in a large bowl.

On top I put a layer of baby spinach leaves, washed. If my farmer's market has really good-looking local spinach, I will buy that instead.

On top of the spinach I put a thin layer of very finely sliced raw onion, either Vidalia in season or a sweet onion from Peru during the winter. This serves as a barrier to keep bacteria from reaching lettuce and spinach, which are the most perishable vegetables I put in my salads.

On top of the onion goes a thick layer of shredded carrot. Next goes a layer of sliced radishes. Then I put small florets of broccoli and cauliflower strewn about.

I use a large plate for a cover and this salad keeps for me all week.

Salad Wrap

When I can't stand the thought of another bowl of salad, I make salad wraps. I put a small bit of a new kind of salad dressing on a large whole-wheat wrap, place the salad such that I can fold the part toward me up over the salad, and fold the sides in over to make a pocket. I can then eat it one-handed while I do my jigsaw puzzle or editing (or catch the latest episode of People's Court!). Nice dressings for this: cheddar horseradish cheese spread, Vidalia onion dressing.

9-Year Celebration of Life

Menu Saturday Aug. 13, 2005

Pico de Gallo *("Peeko day guy-o")*
- tomatoes
- cucumbers
- jalepeño peppers
- onion, garlic
- basil
- salt, pepper
- lime juice

Hinky Dink
- cheddar cheese
- pimento
- sweet pickles
- salted peanuts
- lemon juice
- Miracle Whip

Black Bean Salad
- black beans
- corn
- peppers
- onion
- garlic
- olive oil
- lime juice
- cilantro

Macaroni Salad
- mixed pasta
- celery
- peas
- cucumbers
- carrots
- onion
- Miracle Whip

Mediterranean Potato Salad
- red potatoes
- red onions
- peppers
- salt, pepper
- cider vinegar
- olive oil

Quick Pix
- cucumbers
- rice vinegar
- water
- maple syrup
- onion
- salt

Boston baked beans
Boston brown bread
(both canned, vegetarian)

Assorted breads, crackers & chips

Fruit salad (from Brice)

Iced Tea

9-Year Celebration of Life

Menu Sunday Aug. 14, 2005

Pico de Gallo *("Peeko day guy-o")*
- tomatoes
- cucumbers
- jalepeño peppers
- onion
- garlic
- basil
- salt, pepper
- lime juice

Olive Spread
- black olives
- pecans
- lemon juice
- Miracle Whip

Hinky Dink
- cheddar cheese
- pimento
- sweet pickles
- salted peanuts
- lemon juice
- Miracle Whip

Quick Pix
- cucumbers
- rice vinegar
- water
- maple syrup
- onion
- salt

Tuna Salad
- tuna
- celery
- olives
- onion
- egg, tomato (on top)
- Miracle Whip

Boston baked beans
Boston brown bread
(both canned, vegetarian)

Assorted breads, crackers & chips

Watermelon

Grandma's Potato Salad
- potatoes marinated in
  Grandma's Fr. dressing
- dill pickles
- cucumbers (my addition)
- carrots (my addition)
- celery
- onion
- egg, tomato (on top)

Raggedy Ann Salad

This fun salad was birthday fare at our house growing up. One year we even let the guests make their own! My older sister wanted to have this for her wedding reception, which was being held at our house for just a small group after the church wedding. I'll never forget the church ladies making them all over the various kitchen counters. They managed to get all the Raggedy Ann Salads done and served, to great response! Enjoy them some hot summer day.

Make each salad on a large dinner plate. Be as creative as you want. It helps if you have a picture or actual doll to look at.

shredded carrots (we used grated cheese)	Hair
hard-boiled eggs (slice off bit of back to steady)	Head
cloves	Eyes
piece of carrot	Nose
pimento (from a stuffed olive) (or radish peel)	Mouth
tomato halves cored and trimmed	Bosom (egg nestles in top of tomato)
celery sticks	Arms
thinly sliced ham	Bottom
potato salad	Lower Torso
cottage cheese	Pantaloons (legs)
leaf lettuce	Dress Skirt
ripe olives	Feet

Serve with bread and butter sandwiches, whole grain bread, of course.

We used white bread back in the day, trimmed of crusts and spread with softened butter, two pieces put together with butter as the filling, then chilled. To serve these delicate sandwiches we cut them into quarters (some diagonally and some into "fingers"), stacking them on a plate to be passed around to the guests.

Another memory I have of doing this salad with my mother: I remember her teaching me that the nose is about halfway between the top of the head and the chin, one of my first lessons in an artist's perspective.

Seven-Layer Sandwich

Made and served by my mother as a special tea-time sandwich for visitors — a trifle fancy for just family. Most likely from Irma Rombauer's Joy of Cooking. I have recently resurrected the recipe; it's gotten rave reviews.

Start with a large loaf of whole wheat bread. Trim all crusts. Slice horizontally into four layers of bread, laying them out in order so you will be able to reassemble them the way they originally were.

Before adding a filling, spread bread with mayo or whipped cream cheese (original recipe said butter). Then do similarly with next piece of bread before placing it atop filling. This helps keep filling from soaking into bread.

Start at the bottom of this page (and sandwich) and work yourself up. NOW.

FINALLY, ice all sides and the top of the sandwich with whipped cream cheese. Buy more cream cheese than you think you'll use (approximately 1 lb or 3 C per loaf of bread). Chill sandwich loaf for several hours. Remove wax paper, decorate if desired, and slice carefully to serve. It looks so pretty with all the colors!

Top layer	Top piece of bread. Anchor sandwich with toothpicks to ice.
6th layer	Filling of one of the following: minced chicken salad (with celery and pecans), ham salad (ground ham with finely minced celery), bean salad (black beans, corn or potatoes, finely minced celery, salsa, cumin), black olive/nut salad, tuna salad, or egg salad
5th layer	Second-from-top slice of bread
4th layer	Thinly sliced tomatoes covered with leaf lettuce
3rd layer	Next-to-the-bottom slice from loaf of bread.
2nd layer	Cucumbers, scored and thinly sliced, topped with mint leaves on each slice. Make sure you put sturdiest filling on bottom.
1st layer	Bottom slice of bread from large loaf of whole wheat bread.

To begin, take a large platter, cover it with four pieces of wax paper that overlap in the middle, and assemble the sandwich in the order above. This graphic is upside down from usual order for quick reference when you are making the sandwich.

Wood Man Stew

In the late summer I get reacquainted with my wood man (he's also my driveway man) to talk over plans for the coming months: I heat with a woodstove, and maintain a very long driveway. Recently to our yearly meeting he brought me armfuls of his garden bounty, including a huge bag of beautiful Swiss chard. I say *beautiful* strictly for the esthetic beauty and freshness of the "green," not for any love of its taste or flavor. I must have acted a bit reticent, because Mark began raving about a stew he made with the chard that was so good he could eat it two or three times a week during its peak season. *Sounds like my bruschetta,* I thought to myself. *And pico de gallo.* I had just finished a two-week indulgence in both, with scrumptious whole grain bread.

I glanced at the Swiss chard again. It had dark red stems and huge dark green leaves. It *was* beautiful. Maybe it was time for a change of diet.

Mark proceeded to tell me about his vegetable stew with Swiss chard. "It's like spinach, it cooks way down."

I was skeptical, but that night my friend Brice and I made it. Brice had more experience with chard than I did. "Think of it like a beet without the swollen root. The greens are full of Vitamin A, C, and iron." He showed me how to wash and chop it. "It has more calcium than milk."

Mark was right. It was so delicious I fixed it a day later with another friend, and he asked for the recipe. Here it is.

You'll need a big pot, a large Dutch oven type pot with a lid is ideal. Or a medium soup pot. Put your pot over a medium heat. Add **2 T canola oil or evoo.**

While oil is heating, peel and slice **4 cloves garlic** and add to pot. While garlic is sautéing, peel and chunk **one large onion.** After garlic has softened, add onion to pot.

Stir and cook for a few minutes. While onion and garlic are cooking, prepare next addition, a **medium green zucchini squash.** Trim ends, quarter lengthwise, then cut long strips into man-size cubes, skin and all. When garlic and onion have begun to smell good, dump squash into pot.

Now take a **medium yellow squash**, either summer squash or yellow zucchini, and do the same with it as you did with the squash above, dice into large dice.

Stir mixture in pot, and after a few minutes, add second squash. Prepare **Swiss chard** by washing well each individual leaf, then putting all stems together and chopping off and discarding the last few inches. Chop the stem coarsely, then slice across the chard leaves in bunches. After you have these beautiful green ribbons, give them a chop down the middle the other way, to make the pieces of chard easier to eat. Chard tends to clump when cooked if you don't chop it some, according to Mark. If your chard was especially dirty, rinse in colander after chopping and let drain.

Stir the stew occasionally. When vegetables are beginning to soften, add the chard, a really big bunch, nearly filling the pot. On top of that, put **3 to 4 tomatoes**, trimmed and cut into wedges. Sprinkle liberally with **salt** and LOTS of **black pepper**. Lots.

Put the lid on, let cook for about ten minutes, then reduce heat, stir, and let it cook with the lid on for another ten minutes or so. The chard will shrivel to an edible size, and you will see a wonderful sauce appear (thanks in part to the succulent vegetables). Turn the fire off and let the pot sit for a few minutes so flavors can mingle. Stir again before serving.

Serve in large bowls with chunks of **whole grain bread** on the side, or serve a loaf on a board with a serrated knife so guests can serve themselves.

Mark my wood man was right! It's a simple, delicious stew.

One time I added some cooked black beans as I served it, and it made the stew look really beautiful!

You can add anything you want, or fix it simply as above. Takes 1/2 hour, an easy fix for a busy August supper, when chard is in season.

Mark says this stew is just as good cold. I've never had enough left over to try it cold, though I'm not sure I would have the courage to (sounds horrible). However, I would never have believed in a thousand years that I would ever like or fix this kind of dish, so maybe it is good cold. I'll make more next year. I sure am glad I had someone share the recipe with me. Thanks, Mark!

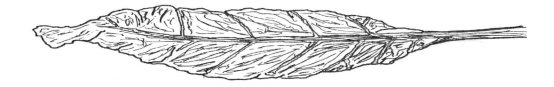

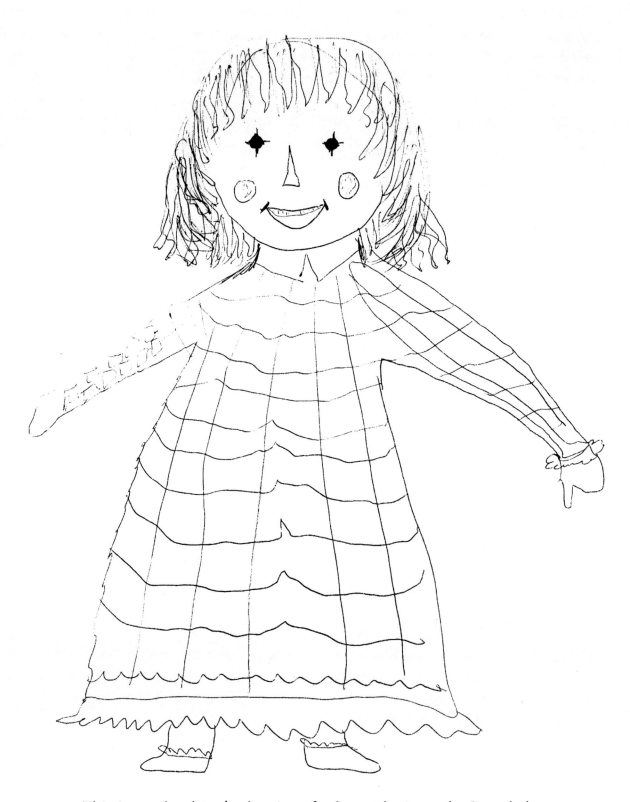

This is my daughter's drawing of a Raggedy Ann cake I made her
when she was 5 or 6 years old.

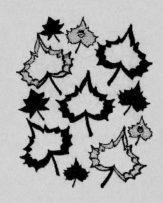 # FALL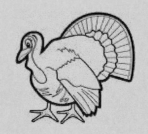

September, October, November

Fall

Fall is the time to enjoy the changing, falling leaves, and prepare for the winter months ahead. Harvest is still in full swing up until frost, with a wide array of squash, potatoes, yams, kale, cabbage, and other fall bounty. Take advantage of what you can purchase locally, from local farmers.

Now is also the time to get a head start by cooking a variety of beans for your freezer. White, brown, red, mottled, black, and everything in between are available in most supermarkets and health food stores. Fresh dried beans cook more quickly than ones that have been sitting around for a long time, so I prefer to get my beans at the supermarket, where the turnover in beans, anyway, is faster than the Amish farmers market where I shop for produce.

Rice is another staple that can be cooked in volume in the fall, then frozen until you want some to go with a stir-fry or curry later in the winter. Potatoes don't freeze very well, especially in large chunks, though if refrigerated, they will keep for long periods of time. Cabbage also keeps well in the refrigerator, as does broccoli. If you don't want to cry, keep your onions in the refrigerator, though Vidalia and other sweet onions cause less of this reaction.

Now is also the time to make some large pots of soup for the winter months.

Don't forget to go look at the changing leaves!

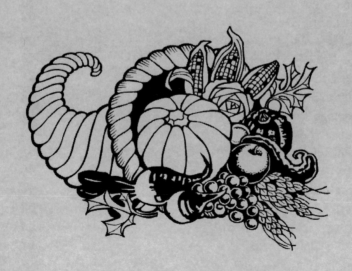

Beans

Beans are very forgiving.

Most bean recipes start out with "soak beans overnight." You can also soak them during the day and cook in the evening. Make sure you have at least two inches of water above the level of the beans to start with. Add more water if necessary to give the beans as much as they want to soak up. Drain and rinse well before cooking.

Cooked beans freeze well. Use pint-size soup containers from your local Chinese restaurant (mine charges me $20 for 50 containers and lids). This size thaws more quickly than anything larger. Many of the recipes in this book use 1 pint (2C) units of frozen beans.

Keep a variety of cooked beans in your freezer. This will give you a healthier version than canned, ready to use in soups, stews, and salads. I keep black beans and pinto beans and a white bean like cannellini or Great Northern in my freezer as stock items.

Cook at least 2 pounds of beans at one time. Each two pounds will give you about 12 - 14 pints of cooked beans. Soak, drain, cover with water, bring to a boil, reduce heat, cook until tender (not hard). Could be 2 - 4 hours or more depending on how old the beans are. Keep a pitcher of room-temperature water near stove to replenish what boils away.

If the beans begin to stick, stir more frequently and add a little water. If beans do stick (like you get a phone call that lasts longer than expected), immediately remove pot from heat and let sit WITHOUT stirring for 10 minutes, then cautiously stir. Beans are done when soft enough but still with substance. You can test by taking a bean or two into a spoon and blowing gently. If skin separates, beans are done. Hard beans aren't good.

If you are too tired to put them away after all the soaking and cooking., leave beans covered until you wake up. By then they will be cool enough to package for the freezer. Fill container with beans using a soup ladle, then add a little of the cooking juice or water just to cover beans. Each pound will make about 7 pints, one for now, 6 to freeze for later.

Beans are a rich source of soluble fiber and have proven themselves in lower levels of colon cancer. People who eat beans regularly adapt to the enzymes produced to digest beans.

Nutrients: B vitamins, protein, low-glycemic carbohydrates, phosphorous and iron.

One of the healthiest starches of non-barcode, natural foods, according to my friend Brice.

Black Bean Chili

This simple chili is always a hit. Use a Dutch oven for double the recipe. Leftovers can be used in a quick quesadilla or burrito.

In a large saucepan heat:

    2 C tomato chunks

    2 C cooked black beans with juice

Add:

    3 - 4 cloves of garlic, sliced

    1 large Vidalia or yellow onion, diced

Stir and cook for 10 minutes, or until tomatoes begin to make sauce. Add:

    2 cups corn (3 ears)

    1 green pepper, diced

Cook 5 - 10 minutes. Add:

    1 T ground cumin

    1 T ground coriander

Taste and adjust seasonings (salt, cumin, etc). If you like it hotter, add chili powder to taste, or hot sauce.

Serve in bowls garnished with a bit of shredded cheese, a dollop of sour cream, or hulled hempseeds.

I like to make this chili in August or September, around the same time I am putting up tomatoes and black beans in the freezer for winter use. Fresh corn on the cob can be shucked, de-haired, and cut off the cob. What you don't use for the chili can be quickly frozen for future use. In the winter, all you'll need is a fresh bell pepper and an onion for the easiest, best chili around. You can substitute canned tomatoes, beans, and corn, but just remember, canned goods were invented to provide survival food for people after a holocaust of war, and were not meant for a healthy diet to rejuvenate or revitalize an adult in the 21st century.

Easy Black Bean Chili

One day when I was feeling especially lazy I put all the ingredients except the spices into a large CorningWare casserole and put it into the oven at 350° until it began to look and smell like chili, then added the spices, stirred, and ate. *M-mm good.* Another time I put frozen chunky tomato sauce and frozen beans in the oven first, and after they were thawed and beginning to coalesce, then added the corn and peppers. After about fifteen minutes I added the spices. This allowed me to continue working until the chili was finished.

Butternut Squash Rounds

Preheat oven to 375°

Scrub **butternut squash** of any size with a brush.

Slice squash across neck and body into 1/2" slices. Remove any seeds with a sharp paring knife. Place all rounds on a large cookie sheet with sides or a large baking pan. Brush with **fresh organic apple cider**. Bake in hot oven for 25 minutes.

Remove pan from oven, baste each round with cider, and turn rounds over immediately (before they have a chance to stick). Brush tops with cider.

Spread each round with a generous portion of the following stuffing and return to oven for 5 - 10 minutes.

This can also be made with acorn squash.

Rice Stuffing

Sauté **1/2 medium onion** in **2 teaspoons hot canola oil**. Add **1 cup frozen peas** and **2 cups cooked mixed brown rice**. Stir and heat. Sprinkle **low-sodium tamari** (a soy sauce) liberally over top of rice. Stir well. Use to stuff peppers or squash.

Seasonal Affect Disorder

Studies have shown that many people naturally crave and/or eat more carbohydrates in October through February — including many carbs that just plain aren't good for us, like candy, cake, white breads, cookies — the sugary starchy processed foods. Why not use intent and choose good carbs? A banana over a candy bar, an apple over a cookie, baked sweet potato over chips, mixed brown rice over French fries?

Carrot Soup

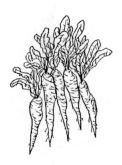

In a Dutch oven heat:

    4 C water

    2 C vegetable broth, concentrated

Add:

    20 large carrots, scrubbed & cut into rough chunks

    1" ginger root, peeled

    1 medium onion, cut into chunks

Cook until vegetables are tender.

Let cool a bit.

Blend in small batches and return to clean pot, or blend with immersion blender.

Add:

    1 to 1 1/2 C almond, hemp, or soy milk

Stir and heat. Sea salt can be added if necessary for taste.

Serve with a sprinkle of **ground cloves** and **a sprig of parsley.**

DaveFest Drizzle

For a number of years my son Dave had a two-day harvest festival at his home called simply "DaveFest." Vegetarian food, vendors with arts and crafts, workshops, and tents for overnighters abounded. One year he even put up an outside shower for the campers. Guests brought and shared food, and because there were people coming and going throughout each day and evening, there were always various foods available.

One of the easiest and most popular dishes I ever took was the following:

On a large platter artfully arrange **slices of garden-fresh tomatoes, slices of scored cucumbers, and basil leaves.** Drizzle with evoo and serve.

Chili Starter

In a medium soup pot or large Dutch oven over low heat put:

4 pints tomato sauce/chunks

1 pint vegetable broth

As these begin to thaw, add:

4 pints cooked beans (pinto, kidney, Roman, black)

When all are bubbly and hot, add the following:

2 C onions, diced

2 C carrots, sliced

2 C celery, sliced

2 C radishes, sliced

Cook until vegetables are tender. If you like it saucier, add a can or two of tomato sauce. If it is too watery, add a can of tomato paste. Cook a bit. Add and stir:

2 T chili powder

1 t crushed red pepper

1 t cayenne or ground red pepper

Take about half out to cool and package in quart-size (at least) containers. Freeze for later use.

To the remaining "starter" (and later, to what you have frozen as Chili Starter), add the following vegetables, as much as you want:

cauliflower, in bite-size pieces

snap peas, cut in two

green beans, cut into pea-size pieces

potatoes, cut into bite-size pieces

Cook until cauliflower is tender. Add last:

bell peppers, in large dice

zucchini squash, in large dice

garlic, smashed and sliced

When all vegetables are done to your liking, serve topped with a bit of **diced onion or scallion**, a little **shredded cheddar cheese,** and a dollop of **sour cream**.

If you want, you can put chili starter in a large casserole dish, add initial vegetables, and let it cook in 350° oven for 30 - 45 minutes. Then add peppers, squash, and garlic for another 15 minutes.

Cornbread

Preheat oven to 425° and prepare an 8" x 8" pan with cooking spray or wax paper (2 sheets, each cut to fit opposite sides and the bottom of the pan).

In large mixing bowl, beat with fork:

     1 large organic egg

     1/2 - 1 C applesauce (or 1 large ripe banana, mashed)

     1 C almond milk

     2 T maple syrup

To this mixture add:

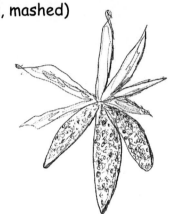

     1 1/4 C mixed flour (various flours)

     3/4 C cornmeal

     1/4 C ground flax seeds

     4 t baking powder

     1 t almond extract

Mix well but not vigorously.

Bake in prepared pan at 425° for 25 minutes.

Remove from pan immediately, peeling off wax paper while bread is still hot.

Serve cut in squares with fruit preserves, maple syrup, or honey. Can be frozen and reheated. Good as a base for vegetarian chili.

Dairy Products

Milk

Cream

Sour cream

Butter

Yogurt

Cheese: cheddar, brie, Swiss, mozzarella, pepper jack, cream cheese, etc.

Amount of calcium is negligible compared to greens such as spinach, Swiss chard, and kale. Eating dairy products increases the likelihood of breast, ovarian, testicular, and prostate cancers.

Mac and Cheese

When you get that craving for macaroni and cheese, or even for that old stand-by of mine, Kraft Dinner, here is an easy, delicious, and more nutritious version that will satisfy your palette. For an even healthier version, add tuna and frozen peas to each layer. This recipe makes a deep casserole dish full. I use an 8" square CorningWare for mine.

Preheat oven to 350°
Heat a large pot or Dutch oven half full of water till it's boiling. Stir in:

> **8 - 10 handfuls elbow macaroni**, whole grain or mixed (about 3 - 4 C)

Return to a slow boil, stirring frequently, and cook until well done (!) not al dente. Drain.

In large deep casserole dish place a layer of drained macaroni. Sprinkle over it:

> a handful or two of **grated cheddar cheese** (≈ a pound total)
> a little **grated mozzarella cheese**
> some **finely grated onion**
> a little **whole wheat flour**

Add a second layer of macaroni, more cheddar, a little mozzarella, a little onion, and a little flour. Add a third layer of macaroni, more cheddar, a little mozzarella, some onion, and a little more flour. Add a fourth layer of macaroni and a thick layer of cheddar. Pour over casserole:

> **1 C almond milk**

DO NOT STIR. Cover and pop into
the preheated oven for 20 minutes.
Meanwhile, mix:

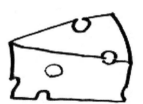

> **3/4 C whole-grain bread crumbs**

with:

> **2 t olive oil**

until crumbs and oil are well integrated. Set aside.

Remove casserole from oven after 20 minutes, take off lid, and spread crumbs evenly on top of casserole. Return to oven without lid for another 10 to 15 minutes or until lightly browned and bubbly.

A casserole that is not deep enough for four layers can be replaced with two smaller deep casseroles, or use three layers if necessary.

Inside-Out Tacos

A new way to eat an old favorite. Be sure and use leafy lettuce as it wraps better.

Brown in a skillet:

      1/2 lb organic ground round

      1/2 lb organic ground chuck

Drain and add:

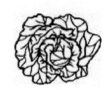

      4 heaping T hot salsa

      4 heaping T sweet pickle relish

      4 mushrooms, chopped

      2 plum tomatoes, diced

      1/2 - 1 sweet onion, diced

      1/2 bell pepper, diced

Mix well and let cook for ten minutes, stirring occasionally.

Heat pre-packaged **crispy tacos** at 325° for 6 - 7 minutes (or 300° for 10 minutes).
Add to meat mixture:

      1/2 - 3/4 C cheddar cheese

When cheese has melted, fill taco shell.

Wrap in 1 large washed **leafy lettuce leaf**. Wrap a second time, reversing second lettuce leaf from first. Lettuce catches dribbles.

Enjoy.

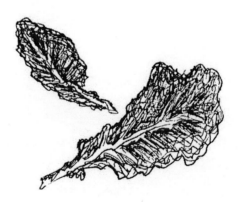

Mashed Yams

I owe the idea for this combination to my friend Brice, who suggested it when we were on a fall Saturday afternoon drive armed with only yams and fruit to eat. We stopped at a little roadside park, gathered wood for a fire, and cooked the yams buried under the coals. A bite of the hot potato eaten with a slice of banana made an exciting new taste. This is my indoor version.

Prick **1 large dark orange yam** (skin will be dark reddish). Bake in 375° oven until fork tender (about 50 minutes). Split in half and let cool for 5 - 10 minutes. Scoop all the potato into a metal or glass mixing bowl. Add **1 ripe banana**, peeled. Mix with electric mixer on low until broken up. Turn mixer to medium and mix well until most lumps have disappeared. Add **1 - 2 T fresh organic cider** and mix well. Enjoy the unusual taste!

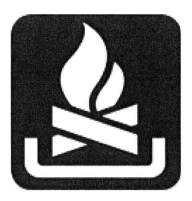

Mashed Yams with Orange

2 dark orange yams or **sweet potatoes**, peeled and cubed
orange juice and **zest of one orange**

Cook yams in water until tender. Smash slightly with a potato masher or hand blender, leaving some small lumps for texture. Add orange juice and zest. Eat with delight. Freezes well.

Mixed Brown Rice

Purchase 4 to 6 different kinds of rice: short grain, long grain, mahogany, basmati, wild rice, etc. Get as much of it organic as you can.

Put all rice into a large bowl or tub. Mix thoroughly. Repackage into pint-size Chinese soup containers, label (I use clear tape and Sharpie for this), date, and freeze.

When ready to cook, bring 3 cups of water to boil in a large saucepan. Add an extra quarter cup of water for the pan. Stir in 2 C (1 pint) mixed brown rice.

When water returns to a boil, lower heat and let rice cook for 45 minutes, stirring on a frequent basis. When rice is done, remove pan from heat, cover, and let sit for 5 - 10 minutes. Stir. Use immediately or cool and package into pint-size Chinese soup containers, label, date, and freeze.

Can be cooked in a large heavy Dutch-oven style kettle in large volume and frozen after cooking.

3 C water	to	2 C rice (1 pint) makes	6 cups cooked rice or	3 pints
6 C water	to	4 C rice (2 pints) makes	12 cups cooked rice or	6 pints
9 C water	to	6 C rice (3 pints) makes	18 cups cooked rice or	9 pints
12 C water	to	8 C rice (4 pints) makes	24 cups cooked rice or	12 pints

Always remember to add an extra quarter to half cup of water for the pan.

I also purchase and cook separately brown jasmine rice, to serve as a change from the mixed brown rice, using proportions above. 2 lbs. rice ≈ 5 C rice to 7 1/2 C water.

I like to make this on one of the first cloudy and chilly mornings of the fall, before the heat is on, and eat a bowl of newly cooked rice for breakfast! Complex carbs like brown rice are excellent for combating the beginnings of winter depression or seasonal affect disorder (SAD), when the sun is out less and less time in October and November. Much better for you than a candy bar!

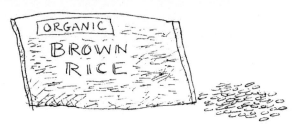

High-Starch Foods

Always eat a low-fiber starch (bananas or yams without skin) with legumes or a high fiber fruit/vegetable (such as berries, broccoli, or kale) to slow down absorption of sugars/starches into the bloodstream.

Eat these foods sparingly (< 10% of diet) and in their most natural state. The less processing a high-starch food has, the more nutrients are retained. Some foods may need cooking to be bio-available (like soy or rice).

Preferable <----------------------	Foods--------------------->	Less Preferable
minimally cooked	Grains	instant or precooked
(oatmeal, brown rice, barley, cornmeal, etc.)		
dark yams	Tubers	light sweet potatoes
skin on (zucchini) or	Squash	peeled or light meat only
dark meat (acorn)		
popcorn, corn on the cob	Corn	canned Niblets
small red with skin	Potatoes	peeled white
		French fries
raw	Bananas	cooked
raw, scrubbed	Carrots	raw peeled, cooked
whole grain	Bread	white, wheat
whole grain	Pasta	white, wheat

© 2009 by Sally Miller

The amount and intensity of color in a fruit or vegetable is directly related to the amount of nutrition: the darker the color, the more nutrition.

Reefer Soup

The day before you shop, clean out your refrigerator and put all your "old" vegetables into a big soup pot along with plenty of water. You can also add a pint of prepared and frozen vegetable broth for additional flavor. Once the water has heated up, turn the heat down to low and let the vegetables simmer.

After an hour, add some frozen or canned tomatoes/tomato sauce. In two hours or so the soup will begin to smell good. Add dried basil and oregano if you want a minestrone-type soup. Salt and pepper are all that is needed, plus garlic.

A typical week that I make this soup is when I've eaten out more than usual, or when some of the long-lasting vegetables like cabbage, celery, and potatoes are getting old.

A typical array of vegetables for me might look like this:

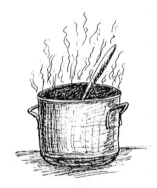

- carrots
- celery
- onion
- potatoes
- snow peas
- cabbage
- green pepper
- broccoli
- lettuce
- spinach

It feels good once in a while to clean out the refrigerator (reefer) completely and start over fresh.

These same ingredients can be blended with a immersion blender for a rich vegetable broth, to be used as a base for other soups. Freezes well.

Shopping Breakfast

Every Thursday my mother used to go shopping, and Thursday for lunch my father finished up the ice cream left over from Sunday dinner. I, too, often go shopping on Thursday, and before I leave, I have a hearty breakfast (shown to keep the impulse buying down).

Heat a medium skillet over medium heat. Add:
> **1 T canola oil**

Add in order shown and let cook a few minutes after each addition:
> **small red potatoes**, sliced (2 or 3)
> **2 carrots**, scrubbed, trimmed, and sliced thickly
> **1 Vidalia onion**, chunked
> **1/2 small zucchini**, sliced thickly
> **1 stalk broccoli**, cut into florets

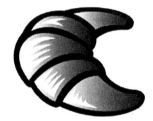

When vegetables are done to your liking, salt, pepper, and enjoy.

Egg and Cheese Croissant

Instead of eating out, make your own breakfast sandwich. Most bakeries and even Dunkin' Donuts carry croissants (well, they carry white bread in crescent-shaped rolls — sigh, for the real puff pastry kind), and croissants freeze well.

When you feel like battering your arteries, remove a frozen croissant, get out an egg, take a small skillet, and put a drop of olive oil on the bottom, smearing it around with your finger. Place on burner at low heat. Scramble the egg with a bit of water in a small dish. By that time the skillet should have heated, and you can pour the egg into the skillet. While it cooks, slice the croissant in half horizontally with a serrated knife. Fold a paper towel in half, place on small plate, and put bottom half of croissant on top of towel. By now egg should have set. With a small spatula fold half of egg onto the other half, so it is now in the shape of a half-moon, or crescent (croissant) moon. Place on croissant bottom. Top with one slice of American or Swiss cheese. Put top of croissant on cheese. Nuke for 39 seconds or long enough for the cheese to melt. Cool and eat.

Stop and Shop Shopping List (in order by category)

Wheat sandwich rolls at bakery. 4 pack (hamburger rolls), loaf whole grain bread, croissants

Batteries, AAA, AA, 9 V, D, C (cheapest, largest package)
Alcohol, H2O2, Q-tips, cotton balls

Water in clear jugs, Appalachian if possible, with handle only

~~Pepsi, Diet 12 pack~~	I crossed these off Nov. 2008
~~Pepsi, Diet, 1/2 size 6 pack~~	after a 60-year addiction to cola, and
~~Dr. Pepper, Diet, 12 pack~~	a 30-year old addiction to aspartame.

V-8 12-oz cans 6-pack
Pineapple juice, small cans 6 pack(s)
Maxwell House coffee Original (mild/smooth)

Rid-X, boxes, White vinegar 1 gallon size; Clorox in handle-able size
Ivory Dishwashing detergent, "classic" scent, large size; Dishwasher detergent "Pure Power"
Pure Power Clear and Free laundry detergent;
Cinch, largest red bottle for refill; Ajax, get Pure Power brand
Viva (Kleenex) paper towel 10+, white only; Vanity Fair paper napkins, "luncheon size"
White Kleenex, "Ultra Soft" only, Regular boxes, Cosmetic size boxes
White Kleenex, "Expressions" for kitchen, yellow/purple/green boxes
White Quilted Northern toilet tissue, double roll only, largest package available

Regular foil, heavy duty (large pkg — long) foil
Handle-tie outdoor garbage bags, 20+
Handle-tie tall kitchen bags (Glad or S&S)
Ziploc bags: gallon size, sandwich, quart, snack, freezer-style 1 gallon, 2 gallon
Contractor bags (huge thick bags, at bottom of shelf)

Wishbone Italian, large bottle
Ken's Vidalia Onion dressing
Bush's vegetarian baked beans
Tuna, canned; 1 chunk, 1 white albacore, both packed in water
Black olives, whole & pitted; chopped or sliced (little cans)
Miracle Whip, glass bottles only, quart or pint
Heinz Sweet Pickle Relish
Wheat Thins, Whole grain Ritz
Dried beans: cannellini, kidney, pinto, Northern, pea, split peas, black-eyed peas, black

I circle what I want, and avoid all impulse shopping.

Amount I save more than pays for helper's time.

Wraps, wheat, tomato, and spinach, Toufayan brand only

Cat food. Large bags Friskies dry food; 12-pack variety pack in cans, variety in cans, get 36+
Brown & Serve Sausages - original, Oscar Mayer Bacon - regular

Amish Farmers Market (in order counter clockwise)

<u>Nuts</u>: Cashews, roasted no salt; pecans, raw; dried cranberries, cherries, raisins,
  jelly, salsa, candy, maple syrup

<u>Cheese</u>: cheddar, pepper jack, mozzarella, Parmigiano Reggiano, Swiss slices,
  American slices, churn butter, sour cream, whipped cream cheese.
  Spices, crackers, dried food, beans, pasta

<u>Vegetables/Fruits</u>: apples, 1 gala, 1 yellow delicious, 1 honey crisp

oranges (big), grapefruit, big, too

squash; butternut, acorn

garlic, shallots, ginger root

Vidalia onions (Peruvian in winter), purple onions

4 small bananas, greenish

1 pineapple

Asian pear, 3 kiwis, clementines

  small red potatoes, brown skin regular size (not baking potatoes), yams

grapes, snow pea pods, jalapeño peppers, snap peas

green pepper, yellow, orange, red pepper

small green zucchini squash

small Kirby cucumbers

1 head cabbage; 1/2 head napa cabbage

1 head cauliflower, no brown

1 bunch spinach (if old, get baby spinach in reefer)

dark or green leafy lettuce, largest head

1 head celery, bok choy if large

rosemary, chives, oregano, basil

  green beans, cantaloupe

  regular mushrooms, sliced, portobello mushrooms (thick not thin)

  4 plum tomatoes, big red ripe tomatoes (in summer only)

  1 pint orange juice, raspberry lemonade, grape juice

  sliced colored peppers, watermelon slice (reddest)

1 bunch broccoli, leeks

2 bunches carrots (think thin) with tops

1 bunch radishes with greenery

parsley, cilantro, scallions (green onions)

tofu, extra firm (check date), garlic

1 bunch asparagus if very thin, peas, corn (by check out)

berries: strawberries, raspberries, blueberries, cherries (by check out)

<u>Meat</u>: ground beef; pierogi

<u>Poultry</u>: ground dark meat turkey, 5 lbs for cats; chicken pies, large brown eggs

<u>Bakery</u>: whole grain bread, oatmeal raisin cookies, molasses cookies, wheat hamburger rolls

> Weekly
> List

> I circle what I want, and how many of each, and teach my helper how to shop for vegetables. I save enough to pay for the help.

Red Lentil Stew

I got this recipe from my sister Martha, who reads several newspapers and clips recipes she thinks I might like and be able to convert into healthier food. This is doubled from the original, with additions to make it a stew instead of a soup.

In a Dutch oven, bring to a boil over low heat (to preserve the nutrients):
>   **10 C vegetable broth/water combination**

Meanwhile, in a skillet heat over low heat:
>   **2 - 3 T evoo** (use canola oil over medium heat if you're in a hurry)

Sauté:
>   **2 C chopped onions**

Add:
>   **1 T each ground coriander, ground cumin, and curry powder**
>   **2 pinches dried cayenne pepper**

Stir until mixture is soft but not brown. Add:
>   **4 large carrots,** halved lengthwise and sliced thinly
>   **5 - 6 small red potatoes,** cut into sixths or quarters (leave skin on)
>   **1/4 head cauliflower,** trimmed and cut into bite-size pieces
>   **6 cloves garlic,** minced

Stir and cook 3 - 4 minutes. Set aside.

When broth is hot, add and stir well:
>   **2 C red lentils** (1 lb), rinsed and picked over

Cook 10 - 15 minutes, more if lentils are old. Add prepared vegetables and spices. Cook 10 minutes, stirring frequently. Add:
>   **4 - 6 mushrooms,** chopped (or 1 rib celery, chopped)
>   **10 - 12 green beans,** trimmed and cut into pea-size pieces (or use peas)
>   **2 medium red or green bell peppers,** chopped

Stir and cook 5 - 10 minutes uncovered, or until lentils are soft. Add water as needed so there is some sauce. Do not overcook. When vegetables are done, add:
>   **1 T vinegar**
>   **1 T maple syrup**

Stir well. Add salt and pepper to taste. Serve in bowls and garnish with freshly chopped cilantro (coriander leaves). For heavier meal, add brown rice. Serves 12.

Freeze what you don't eat. When reheating, add more dried spices as their taste fades. Other colors of lentils (split peas) may be used.

Southern Soup

I first had this wonderful soup at the Veggie Works Vegetarian Restaurant in Belmar, New Jersey. I would never have ordered it myself, but I was dining with members of the Central Jersey Vegetarian Group at our annual fall outing down the shore. I tasted it, and it was delicious! I tried making it myself, with my own ingredients, but it was awful! Then when the Veggie Works Vegan Cookbook came out, I had something to work with (and revise a little). The skin blended in helps slow down the absorption of starches from the potatoes and sugar in the syrup.

In a Dutch oven heat over medium heat:

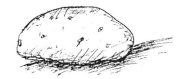

> **4 C vegetable broth**
> **4 C water**
> **1/2 t sea salt**

Meanwhile, prepare:

> **4 large yams**

Brush well under running water. Cut out little bad spots with a small paring knife but leave skin on unless it's really gross. Dice into large dice and dump into pot. Bring to a boil, turn heat to low, and simmer 10 minutes.
Add:

> **1 T extra virgin olive oil**
> **2 T blackstrap molasses or Grade B maple syrup**

Prepare and add:

> **2 cloves garlic**, peeled & sliced

Stir well and cook until potatoes are tender. Add:

> **1/2 C lite coconut milk** (Thai Kitchen or other canned milk)
> **1 t shredded ginger root**
> **1 t lemon zest** (grated rind)

Let sit for several minutes. Blend in small batches until smooth or use immersion blender. Add:

> **1/2 t ground cinnamon**
> **1/2 t freshly ground nutmeg**
> **1/2 t ground cloves**
> **1/2 t allspice**

Stir and reheat as necessary. Add additional coconut milk if soup is too thick.
Serve hot with a pinch of grated nutmeg or chopped cilantro.

Tofu

Open a 6-oz package of firm or extra-firm tofu with a knife, draining liquid into the sink. Rinse tofu well. If you are using only half, cut and put unused portion in a container with a tight top, covering block of tofu with water, to be drained and used another time.

Gently press tofu into a piece of paper towel which you have folded twice to make a square one-fourth the size of the paper towel. Cover with a second piece of paper towel similarly folded. Place all on a plate and put something heavy on top, such as a plate or other object that won't fall off.

Let tofu drain like this for half an hour or more. This will allow the tofu to soak up more of the flavorful marinade or sauce you use.

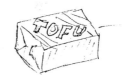

Tomato Barley Soup

I enjoyed the tomato barley soup at a coffee shop in Sycamore, Illinois, on a road trip I took after 9-11. Great to make in the early fall when tomatoes are plentiful.

In a large heavy saucepan (do not use aluminum) place:
4 C tomato sauce
1 1/2 C almond milk
1/2 C water
1/2 C barley
1 carrot, diced (slice in half lengthwise, then quarter lengthwise & chop)
1/2 onion, diced finely
Bring to a slow simmer and cook over low heat until barley is tender (2 - 3 hours). Stir frequently. Add water as needed to make a rich, thick soup.

Serve in a mug with a thick slice of multi-grain bread.

Vidalia Onion Bake

Make this on a cold day to heat your kitchen up, then enjoy this southern version of a quiche!

Heat oven to 400°

In a large skillet over medium low heat:
    2 T olive oil
Sauté until limp:
    4 large Vidalia onions (or Peruvian sweet onions), peeled, halved, & sliced
In the meantime, make crumbs from:
    2 long inner packs (74) Ritz crackers (1/2 of 15 oz pkg)
By hand mix in:
    2 T softened butter or olive oil
Put crumb mixture into a 9" x 12" Pyrex glass baking dish or deep casserole. With back of spoon or fingers (make sure your hands are washed first!) firm crust onto bottom and lower sides of baking dish.

In a large bowl mix:
    1 C sour cream
    1/2 C almond milk
    3 large fresh eggs
    (1/2 C grated Parmigiano Reggiano, cheddar, or Swiss cheese)

When onions are soft, spoon into cracker crust. Pour egg/cream mixture over, and place dish in preheated 400° oven for 10 minutes, then reduce temperature to 300° for 20 - 25 minutes.

Cool at least 10 minutes before serving. Cut into squares (2 1/2" - 3").

I can attest that this is terrible for your arteries! I have substituted olive oil in a couple of places, and almond milk for cow's milk, but it still has lots of animal fat in it. But so delicious!

Almond-Butter Cookies

At the memorial service for the mother of my longtime friend Sandy, I was introduced to a delicious vegan peanut butter cookie (no animal products) made by Holly, Sandy's daughter-in-law. I am so happy that the younger generation is more health conscious than mine. I have omitted two allergenic foods from Holly's cookie recipe. I use almond butter instead of peanut butter and barley flour instead of wheat. You could also use cashew butter.

Preheat oven to 350°

In a large bowl place:

> 2 **sticks soy oleo** (yes, yuck! but it works best)
> 1 **16-oz jar almond butter**
> 1 **C Grade B maple syrup**
> 2 **T water**

Mix well with electric mixer until smooth. Add:

> 2 **C Sucanat** (this is a pure form of sugar cane)

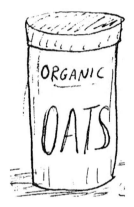

Mix until creamy. Remove beaters and clean them off.
Add to bowl:

> 2 **C organic oatmeal**
> 2 **C barley flour**
> 1 **C oat bran**
> 1 **t baking powder** (make sure it's fresh)
> 1 **t baking soda** (make sure it's fresh)
> 2 **t almond extract**

Mix well by hand. Drop onto large cookie sheets using a large teaspoon (soup size). Flatten a bit with your (cleaned) fingers. Make a pattern by pressing a fork one way and then the other in a criss-cross fashion. Make sure cookies are well separated, as they spread.

Bake in preheated 350° oven for 10 - 12 minutes. Cookies will be quite crisp and crumbly if you let them brown; chewy if you don't. Try them both ways. After you remove cookies from the oven, let cool on cookie sheet for 5 minutes. Remove with a spatula to a double layer of paper towel to cool completely.

Makes 48 - 60 large cookies. Ingredients may be found at most health food stores.

I like to make these just the size to fit into a 4" x 4" Ziploc bag. When all are cooled and bagged, I place them into a larger Ziploc bag for storage in the freezer. I keep these on hand as they are especially liked by the twenty-something workers/friends that help out at the Boxelder Basin Wellness Retreat, as well as by my vegan friends. Sugar is absorbed into the blood stream more slowly with the whole grains and bran.

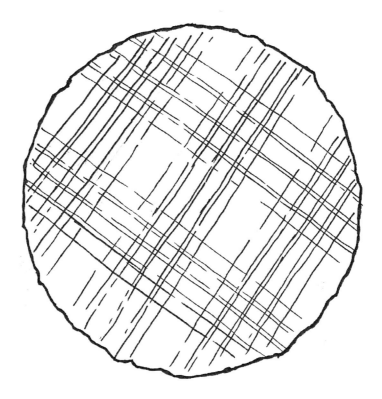

Actual size of cookie.

Recently when I went to make this recipe I forgot that it was double the original recipe and made more than I wanted to bake right then, so I took the unused portion and made it into a cylindrical roll and rolled it up in wax paper. Tucked in the refrigerator, it was ready for the next time I wanted to serve warm cookies with fruit for dessert.

Mock Meatloaf

In the fall when the cool weather hits and you get a craving for meatloaf, try this version, which will fool your eyes, satisfy your palate, and be healthier than meat!

Preheat oven to 375°
Into a large bowl place:

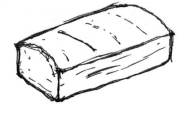

- 2 C cooked pinto beans, mashed
- 2 C finely shredded carrots
- 1 1/2 C organic rolled oats
- 1 C finely chopped spinach
- 1/2 C finely ground walnuts
- 1/2 C tvp (texurized vegetable protein — soy — at health food stores)
- 1/2 large onion, minced
- 1/2 zucchini, shredded
- 3 frozen cubes of tomato sauce, thawed (or 4 T organic ketchup)

For a more refined meatloaf, this version takes more time for food prep, but it has a finer and firmer consistency. Use:

- 2 C cooked pinto beans, mashed
- 1 1/2 C kamut flakes or oatmeal, slightly ground
- 2 carrots, cooked and mashed
- 1 medium onion, finely minced
- 1/2 C fine whole-grain bread crumbs
- 1/2 C finely ground walnuts
- 1/2 - 1 C spinach, finely chopped
- 3 frozen cubes tomato sauce (or 4 T organic ketchup)
- 1 t Worcestershire sauce
- 1 t apricot kernel oil
- 1/2 t sea salt

Mix thoroughly whichever version you choose and shape into loaf on cookie sheet or baking pan. Bake in preheated oven until browned, approximately 1 hour.
Let cool for 5 - 10 minutes. Slice into thick slices and top with lentil gravy.

Serve leftovers in a sandwich with whole grain bread.

Either version can also be made into patties, frozen, and later cooked in a skillet with a small amount of oil. Serve with sautéed mushrooms & onions.

Lentil Gravy

Remember art class in 6th grade? Remember what red and green make when you mix them?

Cook **2 C red lentils** (they look like orange-ish split peas) and **2 C green split peas** in a Dutch oven with **2 C vegetable broth** and **3 C water**. Stir occasionally the first hour, frequently the second hour. Add 1 - 2 C additional water as necessary to keep the gravy from getting too thick. Cook and stir until it is "real" gravy consistency. Add sea salt for flavor. Can be strained or blended if you want an ultra-smooth gravy.

Variations:

Add **green peas** before serving on top of meatloaf.

Add **sliced mushrooms** and cook for a few minutes before serving over meatloaf and/or mashed potatoes.

This gravy can also be used as a sauce for casseroles. Freezes well.

Among vegans there is such negativity towards meat that a mock meat-loaf or a mock turkey is common, and this is one of the reasons I have included this recipe. On the other hand, my belief is that if you don't want to eat meat, you oughtn't to want to eat "mock" meat, either. If you go out for Chinese food, choose dishes with vegetables if you don't want to eat meat. If you order dishes with mock meat, you are only feeding into the "eat meat" mentality. I prefer to eat meat once in a while, buying from a man who feeds his hogs whey and vegetables, no grain at all! And who slaughters them quickly and humanely. I suspect there are other reasons that vegans refuse meat besides the animal rights aspects of it. Of course, for health reasons, it is a good idea to limit what meat you do eat to organic meat, and to small amounts eaten infrequently. As to protein, see page 120.

Tostitos Casserole

In a small casserole dish slightly overlap:

4 or 5 Restaurant-Style Tostitos

Dot with small amounts of:

pico de gallo (recipe page 7)

sliced black olives

cooked black beans, frozen & thawed

Sprinkle liberally with:

shredded cheddar and/or pepper jack cheese

Add a second layer of Tostitos, salsa, olives, beans, and cheese. Add a third if there is room in the casserole dish. Heat in a 350° oven for 10 - 15 minutes, or until cheese is melted. You may want to eat with a spoon and fork. Can be microwaved 2 minutes.

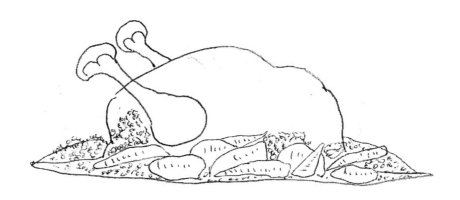

Cranberry Sauce

Cranberries are so good for you!

1 12-oz bag cranberries

3/4 to 1 C raw sugar

1 C orange juice

water as needed

Cook in saucepan over low heat until cranberries begin to pop. Stir, cook until thick, and serve warm. Pour over one sliced banana and/or ripe pineapple chunks for a quick dessert. Serve with Thanksgiving dinner as a relish.

Thanksgiving Squash

Colorful flower-shaped slices of acorn squash filled with a heavenly rice stuffing.

Preheat oven to 375°
Scrub **acorn squash** of any color (or a mix) with a small vegetable brush (not a brush made out of a vegetable, but a brush you have set aside and marked to be used only for vegetables, not for dishes or the sink).

Cut with a large sharp knife across the squash into half-inch slices. Have someone strong to slice the squash if you can't, turning it around while keeping downward pressure. Each slice except the end pieces will look like this:

Of course, you'll want to scrape the seeds out carefully with a small sharp paring knife.

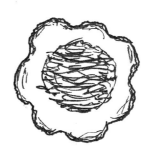

Set each slice in a large baking pan. Brush on a combination of **1 T fresh organic cider** and **1 T Grade B maple syrup** for each squash.

Place in hot oven for 30 minutes. Remove from oven, turn each slice over, brush with cider/syrup combination, and fill with any rice stuffing or the slightly sweet concoction below. Return to oven for 5 - 10 minutes or until squash is just soft and filling is hot.

Rice Delight

To each:
> **2 cups of cooked mixed brown rice**

Add:
> **2/3 C dried almond seeds** (from Oriental store)
> **2/3 C coconut string** (shredded unsweetened coconut)
> **2/3 C lite coconut milk** (Thai Kitchen brand)
> **2/3 C organic raisins**
> **2/3 C uncooked organic kamut flakes** (or oatmeal)
> **1 T Grade B maple syrup**

Stir well and heat. Add more coconut milk if mixture is too dry. Mound in center of squash for cooking as above. Can be used alone as a hot breakfast cereal or as a hot or cold dessert. Freezes well. Particularly nutritious, with high vitamins, minerals, fiber, and taste!

Turkey

The original turkey recipe that I got from my mother started out, singe the pin feathers . . . I doubt if many people today even know what pin feathers are, except Sarah Palin, perhaps! Try and get the most natural, organic turkey you can; fresh is best, but frozen okay. Thaw a frozen turkey in the refrigerator for several days, or in a sink of cold water for many hours, turning frequently until thawed enough to remove giblets and neck from body cavities. Sometimes this can be a struggle if it's still frozen inside. You might as well get a twenty-pound turkey, as the leftovers are varied and it makes wonderful sandwiches! One of my favorite meals, which I allow myself once or twice a year.

Stuff with your favorite stuffing, or my plain one below.

Roast at 325° for 15 minutes per pound — a twenty-pound turkey will take about five hours to roast, and half an hour to sit/set while you make the gravy and cook the vegetables. Don't bother covering, but do baste frequently the last couple of hours. When your meat thermometer registers 170° remove as much of the liquid as you can with the baster to a large Pyrex cup for the gravy. At 180° remove turkey from oven and let rest so internal juices can set. It will continue cooking.

To carve, remove a leg/thigh, slicing pieces onto a serving plate. Make a horizontal cut across the bottom curve of the breast, holding knife point straight into the turkey, perpendicular to the turkey. Then when you slice the breast pieces, they will each end at the cut you've made, rather then tearing in a ragged manner. You'll need a large knife to make a large slice across breast. Keep the skin intact at bottom for later use to cover up exposed meat.

Stuffing

I like to use a bag of commercial seasoned stuffing, adding to it cubes of whole grain bread (about half a loaf) which I have cut and dried — either for a day or two spread out on a kitchen counter or for not too long in a 300° oven. I remember my father making the stuffing at our house.

In a soup pot heat a mixture of butter and canola oil and put onion chopped or diced (depending on how refined you want the stuffing to be), grated carrot, celery chopped or diced, and optional mushrooms chopped. Sauté until golden and add any spice you want (I just use a little salt and pepper, as the commercial cubes are seasoned) and the bread cubes. Mix well.

Pour several cups of hot water over the cubes, mix well, let cool, and stuff the turkey, non-breast side first, then oil bottom of bird and turn over in foil pan. Stuff breast side. Don't put too much stuffing in as it will need to expand, and if it's too tight, you'll end up with a solid lump of junk.

Leave the cavities gaping after you have stuffed, for easier tasting later. Oil the top side. Clean hands are best for this. A very sensual thing to do.

Turkey can be stuffed the evening before you want it, as long as you have some safe place to keep the covered turkey until morning. One Thanksgiving years ago when I lived in suburbia we put the turkey out in the garage, covered with foil, only to find it half eaten by a cat who had squeezed in under the closed garage door! What a disaster that was!

Put it in the cold oven, and it can warm up while the oven warms to 325°. Cook at a lower temperature if you want it to take longer — and especially if you can see by the thermometer that it is getting done faster than you thought, turn the temperature down. Put the meat thermometer in the thick part of the thigh, but if you hit bone, pull it back out some: touching bone will give a false temperature.

Make sure you cook the turkey to an internal temperature of 185 — oops, my old thermometer says, and *Joy of Cooking* says, 190° but they are now saying on the internet, 165°! I don't know what happened during the last 50 years. Could it be that the antibiotics they give most turkeys lower the cooking temperature? I buy Amish and cook to 185. You take responsibility for your own actions.

Gravy

After the liquid you have removed from the turkey pan with your baster sits for a while, the fat will rise to the top. Baste or spoon out fat into a large saucepan, reheat, add equal parts flour or potato flakes. Stir and let cook a bit on a low fire, then add liquid remaining in your measuring cup. Cook and stir. When your vegetables are done, add vegetable water and if needed, some potato water. Continue stirring until it is tasty and smooth. Add salt and pepper as desired. If lumpy, use an immersion blender to smooth.

WINTER

December, January, February

Winter

Winter in New Jersey is moderated by our close proximity to the Atlantic Ocean. We often get a southerly flow of warm air that comes up, and though occasionally it meets the cold flow going across the country and we get snow, more often we get a cold hard rain. Some winters, though, the northern cold dips down further than usual, and we get snow and sub-zero temperatures for a day or two. Brr-rrr, cold! My sister lives in Fargo, North Dakota, and we keep tabs about our respective weather and snowfall in the winter; I don't envy her!

But both of us — along with another sister who lives in Oregon — were raised in Iowa, where the winters, though not as severe as North Dakota, are nonetheless full of much cold weather and snow. Even though I now live in a more temperate climate, I feel the need in the winter to "bulk up" like the squirrels do, and cook food that is heavy on carbohydrates and fat. Fortunately, Martha is much more active than I, and she continues to keep her "girlish figure."

Winter is also a time where I yield to the temptations of the holiday season — first with my Jewish friends, then with my Christian friends and family. After the New Year come birthdays of close friends and family, Chinese New Year, and Valentine's Day, all holidays that have their special sweets.

Heavier but sweeter (more acidic, actually), it's no wonder I'm ready for spring when it eventually comes!

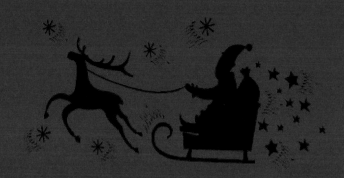

Spinach Tomato Pizza

I like to use a pizza crust made by Vicolo, and I get a package of two crusts at my local health food store. It is made with corn, and is sort of between cornbread and a regular pizza crust. *Mm-m delicious.* One crust is enough for two people.

Preheat oven to 425° and find a large Pyrex pie pan in the back recesses of your cupboards, though actually any large pie pan will do. On top of your crust pour 1 cup pizza sauce. I usually have a pint of homemade in the freezer, but if you don't, you can make a fairly quick sauce from your frozen pints of chunks or sauce. Just simmer on a low heat until thawed and thick. Add garlic, onion, dried or fresh basil and oregano. Stir well and frequently. Let simmer until a bubble coming up blasts onto your stove instead of going back down. That's thick enough.

Meanwhile cut up vegetables. Chop pieces small so they will cook quickly in the hot oven. I often have broccoli, onion, peas, tomato, spinach, pepper, and mushrooms — I try to use at least 5 vegetables. Zucchini squash is too wet to use, yam and potatoes just seem wrong, but almost any other vegetable you like and have is fine.

Put a bit more in the middle of the pie and a little less around the edges, though the Vicolo pizza crusts have a small lip. Top the vegetables with ribbons of spinach leaves and shredded cheese. Probably a cup will suffice — a cup of mozzarella, a little cheddar, and a little pepper jack make it delicious!

Bake at 425° for 20 - 25 minutes. Watch carefully at end. When cheese just starts to brown around the edges, remove pie from oven and let sit a few minutes to cool slightly. Cut with sharp knife or pizza cutter. Kitchen scissors, my former pizza-cutting favorite, don't work very well.

This recipe is the closest I can get to the wonderful vegetable pizzas I used to enjoy in Berkeley during the early eighties. I'd never heard of putting a vegetable on a pizza, but grew to love it. When my children were growing up we even made our own crust at times. Sometimes when I feel like I want a homemade regular-crust pizza, I get some whole wheat dough from my Amish market, and make it as above. You'll never eat another pizza with sausage or pepperoni on it after trying these ideas at home. If you have kids, they'll love making and eating it.

Thanks to Coy for the idea to use fresh diced tomato.

Sautéed Mushrooms and Snow Peas

Heat a large skillet and add:

    1 T extra virgin olive oil

Sauté:

    1 portobello mushroom, sliced

    6 crimini mushrooms (baby portobello), sliced

    6 large white mushrooms, sliced

Add more olive oil if mixture seems too dry as it cooks. As mushrooms begin to brown, add:

    5 cloves garlic, smashed and sliced

    2 handfuls fresh snow peas (sometimes called snow pea pods or Chinese

          pea pods)

    a little salt

    a little pepper

Stir until pods are tender. Serve as is
or with mixed brown rice.

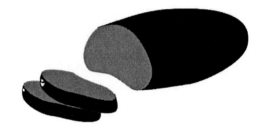

Bread

I learned to appreciate a good bread from my Jewish friends. Thickly cut, heavy — no, dense might be better word — packed with B vitamins and full-fledged carbs, some protein, even more if it has seeds and nuts.

My friend Brice and I used to stop at The Baker in Milford, New Jersey when we were taking a Sunday afternoon drive. When I stayed over at his house the only kind of bread he had was whole wheat, a novelty for me, and The Baker had the best whole wheat and the best whole grain bread around at that time, in the early eighties. Now, of course, many supermarkets have bakeries, and they all seem to stock whole grain bread and rolls. Lucky us!

Gradually I learned to actually prefer whole grain bread after a lifetime of white. My body told me when I had a good piece of bread. Bread is the staff of life, and with bread we can enjoy garlic oil, winter bruschetta, almond butter, and even my newest dietary addition, whipped cream cheese! Do find a good bakery and ask for whole grain bread if they don't have it.

Martha's Stew

This wonderful recipe came from my sister Martha, who found it in The Forum *newspaper (Fargo ND). Of course, I've made substitutions and leave out the chicken from the original.*

Heat in regular-size Dutch oven:

> **2 C concentrated vegetable broth**
> **4 C water**

Meanwhile, scrub with a brush:

> **1 butternut squash** (approx 2 - 3 lbs)

Cut in half crosswise where neck narrows. Peel each half with sharp knife or potato peeler and dice into 1/2" cubes, removing seeds with a spoon. Makes 4 - 6 cups.

Add to water/broth. Bring to a boil, reduce heat, and simmer 20 to 30 minutes, adding during the cooking in order given:

> **1 medium onion,** diced
> **2 - 4 C cooked black beans and juice**
> **1 green bell pepper,** diced in 1/2" dice
> **1 red bell pepper,** diced in 1/2" dice
> **2 cloves garlic,** pressed
> **1 T chili powder**
> **1 T ground cumin**
> **1 t black pepper**

Mix well after each addition. Add water if necessary to allow free stirring of the stew. Sauce should come to within 1" of top of pot.

When squash cubes are tender, add:

> **2 T cornstarch** (or 4 T whole wheat flour) mixed with
> **1/4 C water**

Stir thickener into stew, continuing to stir until stew is thickened, 5 - 10 min. Just before serving stir in:

> **1 T lime juice** (juice of 1 lime)
> **2 T fresh cilantro,** chopped

Serve in bowls with thick slices of any whole grain bread.

Steamed Cauliflower with Crumbs

If you don't have a steamer, buy a stainless steel one with a lid and one or two "baskets." You'll never regret it, even though you don't use it that often in the beginning.

Break cauliflower into florets.
Steam lightly.

Preheat oven to 350°

Mix **3/4 C mixed-grain bread crumbs** (page 18) with **2 t evoo** in a small dish.

Place drained cauliflower in baking pan or flat casserole dish. Sprinkle with crumbs. Heat in 350° oven for 10 - 15 minutes, or until crumbs are lightly brown.

V2: Use broccoli in addition to the cauliflower.

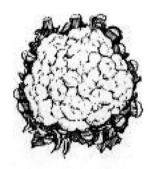

Banana Pineapple Bread

Bake this bread on bad weather days. It warms up the house and you can save on your heat bill!

Preheat oven to 350° and prepare 2 loaf pans with wax paper to cover sides and bottom.

In a large mixing bowl stir together:

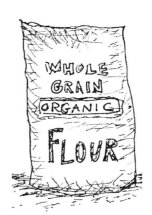

- 1 C whole wheat flour
- 1 C barley flour
- 1 C multigrain flour
- 3/4 C spelt, rye, or other flour
- 1/4 C flax seed meal
- 2 t baking soda
- 1/2 t cinnamon

Set aside.

Blend just until smooth in a blender/food processor:

- 1 C applesauce or apple chunks (previously cooked, frozen, & thawed)
- 3/4 C Sucanat (or raw sugar)
- 1/2 C pineapple chunks (2 rings)
- 6 bananas
- 1/4 C soy milk soured with 1/4 t vinegar
- 2 organic eggs

Pour into dry ingredients and mix well.

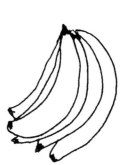

Fold in:

- 1 t almond flavoring (or vanilla)
- 1/2 C pecan pieces
- 1/2 C raisins (or dried cranberries)

Divide into two loaf pans and bake for approximately one hour. Toothpick inserted in the middle should come out clean when done. Cool in pans 5 - 10 minutes with pans sitting on sides to let the steam escape. Loosen ends with knife and remove loaves from pans, pull off wax paper, and complete cooling. Serve warm or cold.

Potato Cauliflower Soup

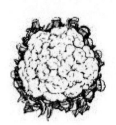

4 C water
4 C vegetable broth
1 medium onion
5 large potatoes
1 small head cauliflower
some cabbage
2 carrots
left over vegetable juice

Cook in Dutch oven over low heat until all vegetables are tender. Blend in batches in blender, or use immersion blender. Pulse if you like it chunky.

Add:

2 C soy milk
salt, to taste

Freeze leftovers for those working days when you don't want to cook.

Potato Cauliflower Leek Soup

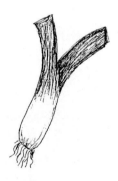

1 qt vegetable broth
4 qt water or to cover
5 lbs potatoes, scrubbed, trimmed, and quartered
1 large head cauliflower, broken into florets
2 leeks, trimmed, washed well, chopped, and rinsed again
2 carrots, trimmed, scrubbed, and chunked
3 C almond milk
salt

Cook in 300° oven until vegetables are tender. Blend well. Add almond milk. If you like it thicker, continue cooking until thickness you like.

Try to include some small red potatoes in your five pounds, as they add fiber to slow down the absorption of sugars and starches.

Potato Carrot Cauliflower Soup

      6 C water (start with 5 C)
      2 C vegetable broth
      3 1/2 - 4 lbs mixed potatoes
      8 carrots
      1/2 head of cauliflower (with stems)
      2 C almond milk

See previous page for methods, one for stovetop, one for oven.

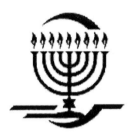

Potato Pancakes

Potato pancakes or latkes are traditional at Hanukkah. These are good anytime!

Preheat oven to warm (below 200°).
Scrub and grate:
      2 potatoes
      1 carrot
      1/2 peeled medium onion
Add and mix:
      1/4 C soy milk
      1/3 C cornmeal
      1 T whole wheat flour
      1 egg (optional)

Heat canola oil in large skillet over medium heat. Drop batter from large oval spoon into hot fat. Flatten slightly if necessary. Fry to a golden brown on one side, then turn over and brown on second side. Remove to a large platter lined with two layers of paper towel. Keep in warm oven until all pancakes are made. Makes 12.

Serve with apple chunks, applesauce, or sour cream.

Sweet Potato Pancakes

I made these potato pancakes one year at Hanukkah for a vegan Jewish friend, and they have been a hit with many others since.

Scrub with a brush:

       1 large sweet potato/yam (dark orange are best for these)

Cut out little bad spots with a small paring knife. Grate potato, with skin on, into a large bowl. Grate in:

       1/2 sweet onion (Vidalia or Mayan onion from Peru)

Make a hole in the middle of your shreds and add:

       1 egg, whipped with fork (leave out for vegan)

       1/2 C soy or almond milk

       3 T spelt or whole wheat flour

       3 T cornmeal

Continue mixing with fork, and slowly incorporate liquid into potato shreds.

Meanwhile, heat over medium heat in a large skillet or Dutch oven (to 1/2"):

       organic canola oil

When fat is hot, use a large dinnerware tablespoon (serving spoon) to scoop out some potato mixture. A fork can help in this process. Carefully lower into fat, flattening with the back of the spoon. Continue to make pancakes, leaving some space between each one. A large skillet will hold five 2" pancakes comfortably; a Dutch oven, four. When pancakes are copper-brown color, carefully turn with a spatula and fork. Cook on second side. Remove to a platter covered with several layers of paper towel. Sprinkle lightly with salt while cooling. Keep in a warm oven (200°) until ready to serve. Add a few tablespoons of fresh oil to pan, let fat reheat, and fry more pancakes, stirring batter before each new batch is formed.

Serve with a cole slaw.

This recipe has slightly more nutrition than sweet potato fries. Makes 10 - 12.
You can also add a little cinnamon, cloves, and nutmeg for a dessert-type flavor. Nice with a fruit bowl.

Quick Sweet Potato Pancakes

Use **1 medium potato, 1/2 onion, 1/4 C soy milk, 1/4 C cornmeal**, and **1 egg**. It's slightly heavier than the one above, but still delicious! Leave out the egg for your vegan friends, though it may need a little more soy milk and flour.

Baked Vegetables

My daughter called me excitedly one night with this recipe she'd thought of, using things she had in her refrigerator. I tried it and it was delicious! Since she is diabetic I was thrilled to see her cooking without sugars or excessive starch.

Glass baking dish
- **asparagus** - break woody end off, wash well
- **carrots** - baby carrots
- **onions** - peel and chunk
- **mushrooms** - sliced
- **tofu** - 1" cubes

Drizzle each of these over vegetables and tofu:
- **apple cider vinegar**
- **tarragon vinegar**
- **evoo**
- **soy sauce**

Cover with aluminum foil and bake in preheated oven at 350° for 45 - 60 minutes.

Squash

Cook whole butternut squash or acorn squash in a 350° oven on a cookie sheet. After 40 - 45 minutes test by pricking with a sharp-tined fork. Cook until almost tender, then remove from oven to cool. It will continue cooking. When cool enough to handle, cut in half lengthwise, scoop out seeds, then scoop out meat of squash. Can be used in soups or eaten as is. Cook several squashes at one time and freeze in pint containers for future use. Do this on cool mornings (or evenings) to warm up the kitchen.

Mushroom Barley Soup

While traveling in the Midwest after 9-11, I had the most delicious mushroom barley soup at the Country Manor Inn Coffee Shop in Jackson, Minnesota, a first for me even though I grew up in the Midwest. This coffee shop was the epitome of a coffee shop from the 40s and 50s, with a simple, friendly style. Coffee shops in the Midwest are the closest to New Jersey diners that you can find if you're on a road trip, or just a local in town, with booths, tables, and always a chili pot and French fries. Extensive menu, standard breakfast, lunch, and dinner fare, includes pork tenderloin sandwich, ham salad on a wheat bun, grilled cheese, club 3-decker, and hamburgers, American fries and eggs of all kind. Fifty years have slipped ethnic additions onto the menu: Reuben sandwiches, French Dip, Taco Salad, and Philly (Cheese Steak) sandwiches reflect today's reality. They wouldn't give me their recipe for Mushroom Barley Soup, so this is as close as I can get to a vegan version (no animal products).

    3 C water (plus up to 1 C additional water as needed)
    2 C concentrated vegetable broth or 3 C regular vegetable broth
    1/2 C barley
    1 medium onion, peeled & diced
    1 C chopped celery, including leaves (wash stalk & cut across all ribs)
    1 t sea salt
    1 t vegetarian Worcestershire sauce (at health food store)
    25 regular white mushrooms, lightly washed, trimmed, and sliced

Heat water and broth in large saucepan or Dutch oven. Add ingredients in order given. Cook over low heat, stirring occasionally, for 2 - 3 hours. Add water if soup gets too thick before the barley is cooked to your taste. I rather like it with some substance, so I often have my first small sampling bowl after the first hour. Adjust seasonings as desired.

The key to a nutritious vegetarian soup is to cook it over a very low heat. Heat kills stuff, as we all know. The hotter the fire, the less life (nutrition) there is.

Black Olive Spread

Drain:

1 small can sliced or chopped black olives

Put into a small chopper. Add:

a handful of pecans, broken or chopped

2" celery stalk (cut across all ribs)

Chop by hand or pulse with miniature Cuisinart (Smart Stick).

Moisten with:

mayo or my favorite, Miracle Whip

Can be used as an open-faced sandwich spread. Use 3 cans olives and comparable nuts/celery for a party. Serve in a small dish with a spoon alongside hors d'oeuvre-size bread and crackers.

Mushroom Hot Wrap

Over medium heat in small amount of evoo, sauté:

1 t ginger, minced

2 cloves garlic, minced

Add one at a time, sautéing each for a few minutes before adding the next:

1/2 small to medium zucchini, cut in 3" toothpick shapes (julienne)

2 scallions, washed, trimmed and cut into 3" pieces

3 thin wedges green cabbage, cut into 3" pieces

1 sliced portobello mushroom, stems cut separately into small pieces

Cook until vegetables are tender.

Heat large burner and warm a large wrap on both sides for just a few seconds to soften it.

Serve the vegetables in wrap, folding so no juices escape.

Berliner Wreaths

Our Christmas cookies always arrived from our grandmother just in time for our father's birthday in mid December, along with our other Christmas presents that we had to wait to open till Christmas Day. This is my favorite family cookie recipe. My sister Martha has carried on the cookie tradition over the years.

Preheat oven to 350°

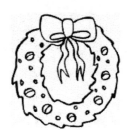

> **yolks of 2 hard-boiled eggs**
> **yolks of 2 raw eggs**
> **2/3 cups sugar**
> **1 cup (2 sticks) unsalted butter** (1/2 lb)
> **3 cups flour**
> **whites of the eggs**, beaten slightly

Powder the hard-boiled egg yolks through a sieve into a large mixing bowl. Mix in the raw egg yolks, and when smooth, gradually stir in the sugar. Then knead in, alternately, a little at a time, the butter and the flour.

Roll out 1/4" thick, using a covered rolling pin and lots of flour to keep it from sticking. Cut into shapes, wreaths being the favorite. If you don't have a wreath cutter, use a 3" biscuit cutter or large glass for the outside cut; cut out the center with a smaller cookie cutter or a sharp knife point. Brush beaten egg whites on the top of each cookie with a pastry brush, then sprinkle with colored sugar. This process is best done by holding the cookie in one hand while painting egg white and sprinkling sugars with the other, all over a plate or the sink. After cookie is ready, place on cookie sheet. (This prevents baked or burned sugar on the pan.)

Martha's technique: shape the dough into a roll approximately 3" in diameter, chill, then slice about a quarter-inch thick. *Beats rolling it out.*

Bake on a greased cookie sheet for 10 - 12 minutes. They shouldn't brown — just the bottom a tiny bit.

Cool on racks and pack in tins with wax paper between each layer.

This recipe is best as is (white flour and sugar). Share them.

Chocolate Fudge Pie

No apologies for this, an old favorite from a cousin on my husband's side who as a medical student actually attended my husband's home birth. This pie was served to us when we visited Dudley and his wife Helen on Staten Island years ago, and it was always a favorite with my kids, who could make it easily..

Preheat oven to 325°

In a metal pan over low heat (or in a microwavable bowl) melt:
> 1/2 C butter (1 stick)
> 1 1-oz square Baker's unsweetened chocolate

Watch carefully so it doesn't burn. Remove from heat and cream in:
> 1 C sugar

Add:
> 2 eggs, slightly beaten

Add and blend:
> 2/3 C flour, sifted (a little less if you use whole wheat)

Add:
> 1 t vanilla

Mix well. Pour into greased pie plate. Bake at 325° for 25 minutes. Middle should be set and pie beginning to pull away from sides of pan when pie is done. Metal pie plate will take 2 - 3 minutes longer than Pyrex.

Serve with vanilla ice cream.

Enchilada Dinner

Using leftover or frozen chili and leftover Cinco de Mayo salad. In a rectangular casserole dish roll up tortillas with layers of mozzarella cheese, chili, and salad. They will be fat. Repeat until casserole dish is full (three for a 7" x 11" Pyrex pan). Lay slices of pepper jack cheese to cover tops of enchiladas, then sprinkle with grated cheddar cheese. Place in a 350° oven for 25 - 30 minutes, or until hot and bubbly. Serve with a bowl of sour cream for those who want a topping.

Roasted Pecans

When I was growing up our mother ordered two cases of pecans from the Shermer Pecan Company in Georgia every December. She made "Aunt Bill's" candy, which took two pounds each batch (and she made ten batches each year to give away as gifts), as well as English toffee, "icebox" cookies, and various others sweets and salads utilizing pecans. I always thought she used so many pecans because she and my father were from the South, and pecans are a Southern delicacy, but now that I am older, I find pecans are far easier on the teeth than many harder nuts like walnuts, filberts, or Brazil nuts.

Preheat oven to 250°

Take two pounds of pecan halves, spread them out in a large baking pan, and drizzle lightly with olive oil (or melted butter if you're not worried about your arteries). Mix with your (clean) hands until all nuts are lightly coated. Wash hands before proceeding.

Place nuts in preheated oven and set timer for 15 minutes. Remove nuts from oven and turn over well with a spatula. Return to oven and set timer for a second 15 minutes. Remove nuts and repeat. The fourth 15 minutes reduce oven to 200° after stirring. In an hour (total) remove from oven (don't let them burn!), dust lightly with salt, and let cool.

Package in cans with plastic bag inserts, then close up plastic and cans. These keep well in refrigerator or freezer and make good gifts in cans you have decorated yourself. People seem to appreciate your efforts.

Just remember, each pound of pecans has 3040 calories, with 80 grams of carbohydrate, 32 grams of protein, and 304 grams of fat.

Each ounce (1/4 C) has:
- 190 calories
- 5 grams of carbohydrates
- 2 grams of protein
- and 19 grams of fat

Rosemary Potatoes

One year I bought a rosemary "tree" at Christmas time and used it as my Christmas tree. I enjoyed snipping little bits of rosemary off and adding them to different recipes. Now I have rosemary growing in my herb garden to use any time! Just before frost I harvest and dry it for winter use. While harvesting and preparing the rosemary I am always reminded of church on Christmas Eve growing up in Iowa. Rosemary is traditionally a Christmas herb.

Preheat oven to 400°

For each person prepare:

> **3 small red potatoes**, scrubbed & cut into sixths
> **3 small regular potatoes**, scrubbed & cut into sixths

Place potatoes in a flat casserole dish. Drizzle liberally with:

> **canola oil**

Sprinkle with:

> **1 T fresh chopped rosemary leaves** (strip leaves from stems first)

Mix well and place in oven for 40 - 45 minutes, or until lightly browned. Every ten minutes or so turn potatoes over with a spatula. When potatoes are tender, sprinkle with a few additional fresh rosemary leaves. If you must salt (try them with no salt first!), use sea salt.

For variation:
After first 10 minutes, add:

> **2 carrots**, scrubbed, trimmed & cut into 2" lengths
> **1 large onion**, peeled & cut into 8 wedges

After first 20 minutes, add:

> **1 small zucchini**, cut into 1" thick rounds

After first 30 minutes, add:

> **1 large green pepper**, cut into 3/4" dice (for method, see page 13)

After 5 more minutes, add:

> **1 T additional rosemary leaves**

This variation can be served as a main dish.

Christmas Ham & Yams

When the ads come on TV for ham just before Christmas, I have found a way to partake in the festivities without overwhelming my digestive system. I purchase a 2 - 3 lb ham slice at the nearby Amish Farmers Market (meaning the meat was raised under humane conditions without hormones, antibiotics, and other harmful substances). I also get a fresh pineapple and organic yams. I make one large pan of food, having one hot meal for myself and a guest. I save a chunk out for a couple of sandwiches, and freeze the rest to have Easter? — another time when I need to satisfy my ham urge. See recipe page 136.

Preheat oven to 350°

In a large baking pan with sides (or a casserole dish) place:
    2 - 3 lb fresh organic ham slice
Score diamond pattern on top of ham slice and insert:
    whole cloves

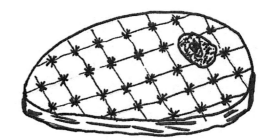

Peel (or not) and cut into 3-inch pieces:
    3 - 4 organic yams or yams
Surround ham slice with yams.

Mix together in 2-cup Pyrex measuring cup:
    1 C fresh orange juice
    1/2 C Grade B maple syrup
    1/2 C molasses
Pour about half of this mixture over ham slice and yams. Place in preheated oven for 30 minutes. Remove pan from oven and baste with juices, adding more syrup mixture as necessary. Return to oven for another 15 minutes. While it is baking, prepare:
    2 thick pineapple slices (see page 76)
Remove ham from oven and place slices of pineapple on top of ham slice. Pour remaining syrup mixture over pineapple. Return to oven for 15 minutes.

Remove from oven, baste yams, ham, and pineapple with juices. Test yams for tenderness. Continue to baste and bake until everything is lightly browned and yams are tender (old yams will take longer).

Make sure and include some pineapple with each serving. Complement hot food with green salad.

The maple syrup, molasses, and yams are full of nutrients. So is the ham if it is organic and natural. OJ and pineapple lose nutrients when cooked.

Christmas Pasta

One year I fixed this for my son Dave and his friend Laura, who came and stayed in my apartment over Christmas for a weekend getaway. Such pretty colors for Christmas time!

> **1 C Amish "dumplings"** or other pasta like bows or Campanelle
> **1 stalk broccoli,** cut into florets
> **2 t extra virgin olive oil (evoo)**
> **6 cloves garlic,** sliced
> **1 tomato,** cubed (I can usually find large Italian or plum tomatoes
>   fresh at Christmas)
> **Parmigiano-Reggiano cheese,** grated

Cook pasta in boiling water until almost *al dente*, then add broccoli to pot. Stir and cook for a minute or two. Save a couple of tablespoons pasta water in a cup or small pitcher, then drain pasta and broccoli in a colander. Do not rinse.

Return pan to stove, add evoo and the garlic (or garlic oil p.94), stirring as it cooks for a minute. Add tomato, let cook for another minute, then return pasta and broccoli to the pan. Add pasta water and a handful of cheese. Let cook another minute, then stir to mix. Sprinkle more cheese in and mix well.

Serve with additional cheese as desired.

This is one of my favorite quick suppers when I'm hungry and tired. One pan is all you need for a meal that's certainly healthier than fast food or frozen processed entrées any time of the year.

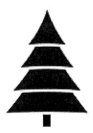

Christmas Toffee

I suppose you could have this a time other than Christmas, but I don't know when. Somehow all the butter and sugar and chocolate and nuts spell Christmas to me. This is an old family recipe my mother learned from her mother, and my sister has been sending some to me for the past 15 years since I stopped making it (sugar feeds tumors most directly). Martha's is thinner and crisper, and she uses chocolate chips. I've tried Hershey bars, but I think this is the best: Baker's German Sweet Chocolate. It's a relatively easy candy recipe as far as candy recipes go, but make sure you have all the equipment and all the ingredients prepared before you start the cooking process. Don't attempt this without a candy thermometer as it is too easy to fail (not enough time at end to test in cold water). Allow at least an hour of time.

You'll need:
- a large heavy pan, at least three quarts. A Dutch oven is fine.
- a candy thermometer
- a large wooden or heavy plastic stirring spoon
- a large slab (marble in the old days) or deep counter from which you have removed everything and that has been thoroughly cleaned and rinsed
- soft butter for "oiling" the slab

Ingredients
- **4 4-oz bars of good chocolate**, broken into pieces for easy smearing
- **1 lb pecans**, finely chopped and divided into two parts (1 1/2 C & 2 1/2 C)
- **1 1/2 lbs butter**
- **3 C sugar**
- **3 T light corn syrup** (Karo)
- **9 T water**

After nuts are chopped (pulse in a blender 1/2 cup at a time), butter your slab (wash your hands, then use 2 tablespoons or so softened butter and smear thickly on slab or counter), ready chocolate into pieces, then start cooking.

Place butter, sugar, light corn syrup, and water in large pan over medium heat. Stir occasionally until butter is melted and sugar is dissolved. When mixture is bubbling well (after about ten minutes), reduce heat to where boiling is continuous but not boiling over, and continue to stir frequently. Change from a slow stir to a faster stir as candy begins to change to a tannish color, foam up more, and thicken somewhat. Temperature at this point is around 240° on the candy thermometer.

At 260° you will be stirring fast, and at 270° you will stir fast constantly as the temperature rises very quickly at the end. You don't want it to burn! *Candy will pull away from the side of the pan and lose its foaminess as it nears completion,* approximately 25 minutes total.

Thermometer should be taken out at 290° and without delay add 1 1/2 cups finely chopped nuts. Stir hard and constantly for exactly 3 minutes. Then quickly pour candy out in a thick, steady stream directly onto your prepared counter (you'll need 24" x 32" at least), using the back of your spoon to spread the candy after all is out of the pan. It is nice to have a helper with this part (if you haven't cried for help before this!). As you spread the candy out, try to make it not too thin, not too thick, and with no holes!

Let pan and spoon cool for later tasting while you space the chocolate squares or pieces out over the entire candy surface. When you get them all laid out, begin, one by one, to move each square slightly, giving it a new place to melt. Keep moving the squares until the entire candy surface is covered with chocolate and all the letters on the chocolate bar have disappeared. Level the chocolate as best you can with your finger or the back of your spoon until all the chocolate is smooth and pleasing to the eye.

Wash your hands well and sprinkle the remaining 2 - 3 cups of chopped nuts over the chocolate surface. Loosen slab of candy all around with a long spatula so it won't stick to counter. Let cool for 24 hours so the chocolate sets well, then remove with a sharp thin spatula, break into pieces, and store in freezer until needed, or put into plastic gift boxes for gift giving. If sending in the mail, leave in larger chunks and place wax paper between layers for slight cushioning.

Good luck not gaining 5 pounds with this recipe!   Christmas 2007

It's nice to have someone to help with this, but it can be done alone. Start out with your non-dominant hand, switching over 2/3 the way through. At that point it gets thicker, and if you switch over, you have your stronger hand to use, fresh and unstrained!

Note from my sister 2008: I finally found my recipe card IN YOUR HANDWRITING; it says spread on a cookie sheet. This was one batch or a third of what you've written this time. I think you should keep the option of using a cookie sheet since it is much more "available" than a suitable counter surface. I'd be afraid of burning my laminate counter. Plus the sheet is easy to move when done, to a cool place or even the refrigerator if in a hurry to cool and set. And it doesn't need to be buttered before spreading.

Dave M, one of my assistants, made a batch with a thick bottom, dark chocolate, and crushed candy canes on top. Pretty and delicious! He put a few pieces in small Ziploc bags (3x4) with his sticker tags, and gave these small tokens of his appreciation to his paper route and candle customers at Christmas.

Cranberry Pineapple Dessert

Often cranberries and pineapple are plentiful in the weeks surrounding Thanksgiving and Christmas. If you find yourself with ample of both, try this scrumptious dessert that is grand enough to take to a party.

Make sure you let the fresh cranberries and whole fresh pineapple ripen — the pineapple on the kitchen table and the cranberries in the refrigerator. Ripe fruit makes a decidedly better dessert.

Preheat oven to 350°

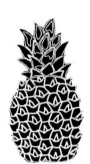

Melt on top of stove or in oven in a 10" x 15" baking pan:

    1/2 C (1 stick) soy margarine (or butter)

Add:

    2 C fresh cranberries, washed and picked over

    1 C Sucanat (a brownish sugar in pure form)

    1/2 C apple cider (or grape juice)

Stir until well mixed and berries are slightly softened, 5 - 10 minutes. Remove from heat and even out cranberries over entire pan. Top with:

    6 - 10 slices of fresh pineapple, peeled and cored

Perfect Pineapple Prep

Let a fresh pineapple sit on your counter, out of the way, to ripen; and when you come into the kitchen sometime and smell it, you'll know it's ripe. Fruit ripens to attract us, and ripening sweetens the fruit, which attracts babies to like it (they have sweet buds to attract them to sweet fruit rather than sour, unripe fruit).

If using a whole pineapple, "top and tail" the pineapple and discard same. For rings, slice the thickness you want, slice off outer skin/peel, and remove core from each slice with a sharp paring knife. For chunks, split pineapple across the middle, peel each half with knife, cut each half into quarters, cut out core on each quarter, then cut each into long spears, then into chunks.

If pineapple is large or you want to use only half, use lower half first as it ripens earlier. First cut off tail, then bottom half, and put top half, with top intact, on a plate and refrigerate for later use (it will keep a week or so). Treat lower half as above, for use as rings, spears, or chunks.

In the meantime, place in a large mixing bowl:

      1 white cake mix

      1 1/4 C water (or juice)

      1/4 C applesauce (or mashed banana)

      2 eggs (not necessary, but better with than without)

Mix with electric mixer for 2 minutes.

Add:

      1 C fresh ripe cranberries, washed and picked over

Mix for 2 more minutes, scraping sides of bowl.

Remove beaters and fold in:

      1 C pecan pieces (or walnut pieces)

Spoon out stiff cake batter onto top of prepared fruit in pan, spreading almost to the edge of the pan.

Bake in 350° preheated oven for 40 - 45 minutes, until top is deep golden brown. Test for doneness by sticking a skewer or toothpick into cake in the middle of the pan. If it comes out clean, it's done. If it's dough-y, give it a little longer to cook.

Remove from oven and let cool for 5 - 10 minutes, or until top edge of pan is warm but not hot to the touch. With a table knife loosen sides of cake from pan. Place large rectangular tray (11" x 16") on top of the cake pan, upside down. Using 2 oven mitts or heavy towels, quickly invert tray and pan together, holding tight so mixture won't leak. As an additional precaution, flip over sink or clean counter. Do this step with confidence!

Let the pan sit on top for a few minutes to cool additionally and let cake fall completely onto tray. You may need to lift a corner of the pan with a fork to let the steam escape.

Elegant and delish! Can be served warm or cold.

Substitute disposable lasagna pan or any shape deep pan as long as you have a similar tray or large plate to hold the finished cake(s).

Serves 24

Arnie's Birthday Menu   January 8, 2005

The Central Jersey Vegetarian Group gave a surprise fiftieth birthday dinner for one of its most loyal members, Arnie Kushnick, at an Asian fusion restaurant in Rocky Hill NJ. Stacey, the founder and president of CJVG, and I brought dessert. It was a wonderful event, and Arnie was surprised right up to the last. We included many of his old friends from around the New York area.

Appetizers
> Vegetable Dumplings, steamed and fried
> Spring rolls
> Cucumber w/garlic
> Scallion pancakes

Soups
> Hot and Sour
> Vegetables & Bean Curd

Entrees
> Sautéed Taiwanese baby cabbage
> Sautéed Chinese broccoli
> Spinach with fresh garlic
> Snow cabbage, bean curd sheet, and pea pot
> String beans in brown sauce (spicy)
> Moo Shu Vegetables w/pancakes
> 3 Musketeers (beans, asparagus, and snow peas in a white sauce)
> Long Life Vegetarian (steamed vegetables) w/garlic, white sauce on the side
> Thai Silver Noodles (no egg, hot and spicy)
> Vegetable Lo Mein

Brown rice

Desserts
> Chocolate pan pie
> Cranberry Pineapple dessert (p.76)

Tea

Menu items contain no MSG, egg, meat, chicken broth, milk, or other dairy.

Winter Rice

My young helper Brian, a chef at his other job, first showed me how to make cranberry sauce with fresh cranberries. I could never go back to canned cranberry sauce, and I have found many other ways to use this versatile fruit.
These are two of my favorites.

In a large saucepan stir together:

     1 C fresh cranberries

     1 12-oz jar fruit preserves (sweetened with fruit juice)

     1/3 C orange juice

     1/4 C Sucanat

Stir and cook over slow heat until jam is melted and cranberries begin to pop. Cook until thickened, then stir in:

     1/2 fresh pineapple, cut into small chunks (≈ 2 1/2 C)

     1 C raw or roasted cashews

Add to this mixture:

     3 C cooked mixed brown rice (1 C uncooked)

Stir until warm, and serve.

Pecan Rice

Sauté for 3 - 4 minutes in a small amount of olive oil:

     1/2 Vidalia onion, chopped

     1 carrot, shredded

     1 C fresh or frozen peas

Add:

     2 thick rings fresh pineapple, cut into small bite-size pieces

     1 C pecan halves

     1/2 C dried cranberries

     1 T sesame seeds

     1/4 C apricot preserves

     1/2 C hoisin sauce

Stir until hot and mixed. Add:

     2 C brown rice

Mix and enjoy.

Both of these dishes can be served as a dessert, a side dish, or a light meal.

Vegan Chocolate Birthday Cake

I created this for my son Dave's 41st January birthday (his 40th got snowed out!) The original cake came from my vegan friend Arnie, who found the original recipe in Fran Costigan's Good Desserts.

Preheat oven to 350°

In large bowl mix together:

- **3/4 C whole wheat flour**
- **3/4 C barley flour**
- **3 T + 1 t cocoa powder**
- **2 t baking powder**
- **1/2 t cinnamon**
- **1/2 t sea salt**
- **1/4 t baking soda**

Set aside. In a 4-cup Pyrex cup mix well with a whisk:

- **1 C Grade A maple syrup**
- **1/2 C vanilla almond milk**
- **1/4 C canola oil**
- **1/4 C water**
- **1 1/2 t apple cider or white distilled vinegar**
- **1 t almond extract**
- **1/2 t vanilla**

Pour liquids into dry ingredients; mix well. Spoon into muffin tins lined with paper baking cups. Makes 12 large cupcakes (to be split after baking) or 24 thinner ones (which can be used as layers). Bake for 18 - 20 minutes. Watch the cakes rise, set (like eggs do), look dry, and each will spring back at center when touched lightly near the end of baking time. A toothpick or tiny skewer will come out clean when inserted in the middle.

Batter can also be made into 2 round layers, baked for 25 - 30 minutes in pans that have been oiled, floured, and shaken out. For a larger crowd (24) make a double recipe and use two 9" by 13" pans (each will be one layer).

Cool all size cakes completely before filling. All sizes can be baked ahead and frozen for later assembly (the 9" x 13" is hard to handle, but as Arnie says, *if it breaks, you can always fill in the cracks with icing or pudding*).

For filling use:
- **whole cherry preserves sweetened with fruit juice** (1 pint)
- **vegan chocolate pudding** (double the recipe for 9" x 13" cake, or make 2x)

Vegan Chocolate Pudding

I remember making chocolate pudding as a child with my mother. After it had thickened, we filled our (always) clean sink with cold water, an inch or so, and put the pudding pot in the middle. One of my first "hot food" jobs was to stir the pudding while it cooled, being careful not to let the faucet drip into the pudding. When it was cool to the touch of your finger (of course, you got to lick after testing), we would pour it into individual pudding bowls, refrigerate, and enjoy for dessert. This recipe is even better, and healthier, though it still has many carbs and calories!

In small bowl dissolve:

4 T cornstarch

In:

1/4 C almond milk

Set aside, but keep a spoon nearby so you can give it a stir before you use it.

In double boiler or a bowl over hot water melt:

1 square Baker's unsweetened chocolate (1/4 C semi-sweet chocolate chips)

Stir in:

1 1/2 C vanilla-flavored almond milk

1/2 C Grade A maple syrup

Heat and stir until just to, but not yet boiling (steam will come up from pot). Slowly add cornstarch mixture. Cook and stir over hot water or *very* low heat until thickened.
Continue cooking and stirring for 5 - 10 minutes, or until thicker. Don't be impatient. Cool off the stove. Stir in:

1/2 t almond extract

Makes 4 1/2-cup servings.

For pudding, spoon over cup-up fruit, such as bananas, apples, or orange segments, in small bowls.

To assemble cake, split each cupcake and spread a layer of cherry preserves on the bottom layer. Put a layer of cooled pudding on top of cherry filling, replace top of cupcake, and add layer of pudding on top of cupcake instead of icing. Serve each on a small plate topped with a birthday candle. Finish other cakes in a similar way. Used as a cake filling and icing, the pudding, though thick and cool, tends to run down cake sides and split after refrigeration for more than 4 - 5 hours, so ice near serving for best results.

Fruit Pancakes

In the winter our bodies crave extra carbohydrate to compensate for the lack of sunlight. Though beans are a healthier choice, some days pancakes just hit the spot. These are a little healthier (and cheaper) than IHOP.

Use a **whole-grain pancake mix.**
Heat griddle and add thin coating of canola oil.
In large Pyrex cup place:

> 1 1/2 C mix
> 1 egg
> 1 1/4 C almond milk.

Stir and add three or four of the ingredients below:

> 1 **banana,** sliced
> 1/2 C **blueberries**
> 1/2 C **strawberries,** sliced
> 1/2 C **pineapple chunks**

Stir gently. When griddle is hot (a drop of water sizzles and dances around), make a small test pancake in the middle of the griddle. When bubbles pop and *stay open*, flip pancake and cook on second side. Keep warm and make the rest of the pancakes. Add almond milk if too thick. Freeze leftover pancakes.

Serve with Grade A maple syrup or fruit preserves.

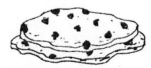 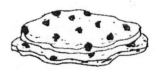

Winter Salad

In the winter I like to make up a big bowl of this salad to keep in the refrigerator so I can have a ready-made side to cooked food (my predilection in winter). The red cranberries provide an interesting winter change.

1 large red apple (delicious, gala, or honey crisp)
1 large yellow delicious apple
celery
walnut or **pecan pieces**
dried cranberries or **cherries** (I get unsweetened ones from my Amish
    market)
mayonnaise or my favorite, **Miracle Whip**

Dice apples and celery, add nuts and berries, mix well with salad dressing. Chill. Mix well and serve on individual plates atop a bed of leafy lettuce and baby spinach.

There are no amounts with this recipe as your taste will vary from time to time. I usually let my inner nutritional needs dictate how much celery, nuts, or dried fruit to use.

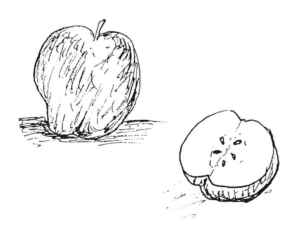

The more efficient you are in your food preparation,
the more time you have to talk with your family and
guests, watch TV, or enjoy the silence while you eat alone.

Chinese New Year

Chinese New Year usually falls at the end of January/beginning of February, and one year the Central Jersey Vegetarian Group had a Buddhist banquet, which Li Chung arranged at the Opera House Chinese Restaurant in Rocky Hill, New Jersey. We were served a selection of authentic Buddhist food which was also vegan, contained no garlic or onion, and was also wheat free.

Prepare and add to a large-size steamer over gently boiling water, in order given below:

      1 large sweet potato/yam, peeled & cubed
      2 carrots, trimmed, scrubbed & cut into 1" thick rounds
      1/3 head cauliflower, cut into 1" pieces
      1/4 head green cabbage, chopped
      1/4 head napa, (Chinese cabbage), chopped
      10 - 12 green beans, trimmed & cut into 1" pieces
      10 - 12 pea pods, cut in half

When vegetables are done to your liking, transfer to a large serving dish and add approximately **1/2 8-oz jar hoisin sauce** over the top of vegetables. Serve with mixed brown rice.

Buddhists eat no garlic, onion, chives, radishes, or leeks because these "five spices" tend to excite the senses. Since I have "Surplus Attention Syndrome," or SAS, I *love* to have my senses excited! But seriously, I do use garlic and onion as mild antibiotics, and radish to reduce gall bladder distress. One radish eaten in small bites, thoroughly chewed, on an empty stomach before meals will help reduce a gallstone which is giving you problems. One radish a day maintenance will keep a gallstone at bay. Garlic and onion raw are always good additions to the diet when you have over-imbibed in dairy or meat.

Oriental Dumplings

I am making these dumplings in the front cover picture.

> **1/4 head green cabbage** (preferably Korean or Taiwanese), finely chopped
> **1/4 head napa** (Chinese cabbage), finely chopped
> **2 handfuls spinach**, chopped
> **2 mushrooms**, finely chopped
> **1 carrot**, shredded
> **1/2 Vidalia onion**, finely minced
> **1/2 C peas** (or green beans, chopped)
> **1" ginger root**, peeled, then shredded or finely minced
> **1 T hoisin sauce**
> **1 t water**

Cook ingredients in large saucepan or Dutch oven, adding one at a time in order given. Add ginger and hoisin sauce. Stir well, cooking until reduced in volume. Using pre-made round dumpling wrappers, put a small amount of filling off center, then dip finger into little dish with water in it and go around edge of wrapper. Fold in half around filling, pressing edges together. Place on sheet of paper towel to set up for cooking (at least 1/2 hour).

Preheat electric skillet to medium hot (350°) and add 1/2" canola oil. Fry on one side, then remove to clean paper towel. Alternatively, fry on both sides in smaller amount of oil. Or healthier yet, steam dumplings in steamer for 5 minutes. Keep warm until ready to eat, though they don't keep well for long periods of time. Serve with sauce made with: **1/3 C each hoisin sauce, water,** and **chopped scallion,** or try sauce below.

Apricot Scallion Sesame Sauce

Can be used on a Chinese pancake for Moo Shu, as a sauce for stir-fry, or with spring rolls.

Sauté in canola oil over medium high heat:
> **2 bunches of scallions,** trimmed & chopped
> **2 - 5 cloves of garlic,** minced

When toasted on edges, add:
> **2 T sesame seeds,** white, black or mixed

Toss for a half minute or so. Reduce heat and add:
> **1 12-oz jar apricot preserves,** sweetened with juice

Stir frequently. Once liquefied to a syrup, add:
> **1 8-oz jar hoison sauce,** vegetarian with sweet potatoes if possible

Bring to a simmer and serve warm. Wonderful with tortilla chips. Keep in refrigerator.

Vegan Valentine's Day

Menu

Steamed Cauliflower with Crumbs (p.60)

Portobello Burgers on Whole Grain Rolls (p.9)
    tomato, dill pickle slices, baby spinach leaves, lettuce
    condiments as desired (ketchup, mustard, etc.)
    cooked or raw onion

Vegan Chocolate Pie with Bananas (p.81)

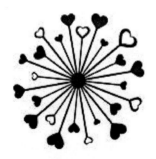

Winter Vegetables

After a cold sunny afternoon out running errands, I like nothing better than to put a pan of root vegetables into the oven to cook while I get a fire started in the woodstove and put my feet up for a few minutes. Rachael Ray, from whom I got this recipe, does it in less than 30 minutes. Mine always seem to take longer.

Preheat oven to 400°

In a 9" x 13" baking pan, place the following vegetables:

10 - 12 little red potatoes, cut into quarters or sixths

10 - 12 baby bella or crimini mushrooms, halved

3 large carrots, scrubbed, trimmed & cut into 1" chunks

1 large Vidalia onion, cut into 1" chunks

1 small sweet potato or yam, peeled & cut into 1" chunks

1/2 turnip or rutabaga, peeled & cut into 1/2" chunks (these are strong flavored, so go easy until you know you like them)

Mix by hand. Add:

1 - 2 T extra virgin olive oil

leaves from 2 branches fresh rosemary, chopped

Mix well. Place in preheated oven for 30 - 60 minutes, or until tender, turning vegetables over with a spatula every 15 minutes.

Can be used as a side dish or eaten as a main dish with a Waldorf (apple) salad to complement.

I can't believe Rachael Ray actually still peels her carrots! Scrub with a vegetable brush and save some nutrients!

Winter Bruschetta

When tomatoes are out of season, this is a nice little Italian appetizer to serve. Great for a quick breakfast, too! You can use frozen beans if you have them.

Soak overnight or for at least 8 hours:

1 C cannellini beans (or other white bean, such as Great Northern)

Rinse well. Place in medium saucepan and add:

2 C water

2 C vegetable broth

Bring to a boil, reduce heat to low, and cook until tender, 2 - 3 hours. Check water/broth level frequently after 1 1/2 hours and make sure there is plenty of liquid. Add water as necessary to cover beans.

While beans are cooking, prepare toast. Use **whole grain bread.** A long skinny loaf is preferable, but small whole grain rolls will do. Cut into 1/2" slices and arrange slices on a cookie sheet. Drizzle or brush with **extra virgin olive oil.** Put under broiler, watching carefully, until lightly browned. (Toaster oven can be used for small amounts of toast.) Remove from heat and put toasted side down on oven proof serving dish. Bread can be toasted on both sides if you like a crispier toast, but it's harder to eat.

Nutrition Highlights of Beans and Chicken

1 C Great Northern beans (177g) (boiled)
Calories: 209
Protein: 14.7g
Carbohydrates: 37.3g
Total fat: 0.7g
Fiber: 12.4g

1 C chicken breast (140g) (roasted)
Calories: 231
Protein: 43 g
Carbohydrate: 0
Total Fat: 5g
Fiber: 0

Beans are an excellent source of: Iron (3.7mg), Magnesium (88.5mg) and Folate (181mcg)
Foods that are an "excellent source" of a particular nutrient provide 20% or more of the recommended daily value.

Beans are a good source of: Calcium (120mg)
Foods that are a "good source" of a particular nutrient provide between 10 and 20% of the recommended daily value.

When beans are tender (or thawed if you're using frozen), add to pan:

1 C water or broth

Mash bean mixture with back of fork (or pulse with an immersion blender) and add:

8 cloves of garlic, smashed

1 t dried oregano

1 t dried basil

salt and pepper

Continue to stir and cook until well mixed, thick, and somewhat smooth.

Spread bean mixture onto toast slices. Top with:

grated Parmigiano-Reggiano cheese

Just before serving place under broiler until cheese melts. Cut large bread slices in half before serving.

Beans and toast can be made ahead of time. Beans keep in refrigerator for a day or two, and both beans and cheese freeze well. Parmesan from the supermarket won't do. Get Parmigiano Reggiano at a specialty cheese or Italian store and grate it yourself.

In general it's better to add vegetables to a stew, curry or stir-fry one at a time, giving each a few seconds to warm up on top before folding in.

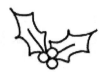

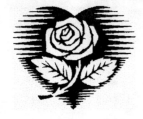

SPRING

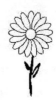

March, April, May

Spring

Spring in nature is a time of increasing light, increasing warmth, increasing movement: a time of birth and rebirth. Perennials begin to show in the garden, trees and shrubs bud, birds nest, and peepers call out danger when animals come to feed in the wetlands.

Berries are plentiful for feeding our freezers and enjoying fresh. Lettuces and other cool weather foods like carrots, spinach, and peas grow and begin to mature.

For me it is a time for housecleaning — not just the clutter that has accumulated in the actual house, but also the clutter my body has accumulated over the long winter. In many people "colds" abound, which is nature's way of cleaning out all that body clutter.

Before the onslaught of spring mania, treat your body with dignity. Cut WAY back on cheese and meat to allow your body time to rejuvenate itself without the undue pressures of heavy digestion. If you don't, you may find yourself coughing and blowing and coughing some more.

Many of the recipes in this section take advantage of spring foods, and support spring cleaning, to ready our bodies for increased activity. We are, of course, part of nature.

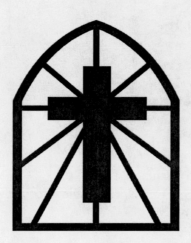

Spring Thing

In the spring, especially after a winter of relative inactivity and of eating indiscretions, it's a good thing to give your body natural cleansers like garlic, hot peppers, curry, ginger, and onion. Use all of these as close to raw as you can stand, as in their raw state they are anti-biotic *for those bad critters feeding on your misadventures.*

Heat a Dutch oven or large saucepan over medium low heat. Add:

> **2 T extra virgin olive oil**

Sauté in order given:

> **3 scallions,** chopped
>
> **1 T minced ginger**
>
> **3 cloves garlic,** smashed and minced
>
> **4 large regular mushrooms,** sliced
>
> **4 crimini** (brown or baby portobello mushrooms), sliced
>
> **2 portobello mushrooms,** sliced then cut in half if they are large

If mixture appears too dry, drizzle on another tablespoon olive oil.
Add and sauté:

> **1/2 head green cabbage,** quartered, cored, and thinly sliced
>
> **1 carrot,** shredded

When cabbage is wilted (5 - 10 minutes), add:

> **3 T hoisin sauce** (or sauce on page 85)
>
> **1 T water**
>
> **3 additional cloves garlic,** smashed & minced

Lower heat and stir well.

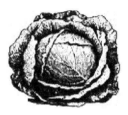

Serve with mixed brown rice in large bowls.

Stir-fry Asparagus

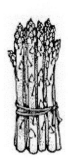

Heat olive oil in large skillet or wok over medium heat. Add:

   6 cloves garlic, sliced

Peel, halve and slice thin:

   1 Vidalia onion

Add to skillet and stir with spatula or shake. Add:

   4 - 6 mushrooms, sliced

Stir and let cook a bit. Meanwhile, wash well:

   1 bunch asparagus

Break one or two spears near stem end (below this it gets woody and difficult to chew). Line these natural breaks up. Place rest of asparagus with tip ends lined up, and cut across entire bunch at one time to line up with ones broken. Discard stem ends. Wash remaining asparagus well and chop into 1" lengths.

Add to skillet all asparagus pieces except dainty tips. Save them for a few minutes, then add to stir-fry. Use spatula to keep vegetables moving. When asparagus turns color to a bright green and is as tender as you like it, remove all to a serving bowl and enjoy!

Asparagus Omelette

Fix asparagus as above. Remove to serving plate. Break 4 eggs and scramble with a fork, adding about 2 teaspoons of water. Pour into skillet over low heat. Let eggs set.

When almost cooked on top, add half of asparagus onto one side of eggs. Flip other side of the omelette over onto asparagus side, carefully. Remove all to serving plate and top with remaining asparagus. For well done, nuke for 39 seconds.

Shrove Tuesday Dinner (to use up fat in the house before Lent)

   Carrot Soup with Cloves (p.32)
   Steamed Broccoli and Cauliflower with Crumbs (p.60)
   Potato Pancakes w/Applesauce & Sour Cream (p.63)
   Chocolate Almond Pudding with Bananas (p.81)

92

Hot and Sour Soup

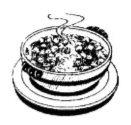

In a Dutch oven heat:

4 C water

Into water drop frozen blocks of:

2 C vegetable broth

2 C clear (strained) **vegetable broth**

When broth is thawed and mixture is just under a boil, turn heat down to medium low and add to broth in order given:

1 carrot, cubed

1 package extra firm tofu, cut into 1/3" cubes

10 - 12 green beans, slivered & cut in half

10 - 12 snow peas, slivered & cut in half

10 - 12 small cauliflower florets

10 - 12 small mushrooms, trimmed & sliced (leave stem on)

3 - 4 scallions, trimmed & cut across both white and green parts

1 t hot pepper flakes

1 t dried lemon grass (get at Asian store)

Put the lemon grass in cheese cloth or retrieve before serving.

Simmer until cauliflower is tender. Just before serving add:

1 T tamari sauce

juice from one lime

Adjust seasonings as desired.

Juicing Limes or Lemons

Roll room-temperature lime or lemon, cut in half not through stem end, poke holes into flesh of lime with a fork, remove any seeds, and squeeze into small cup or bowl before adding to soup. Use 1 lime for 1 T of juice; 1/2 lemon gives 1 T.

Bowls

Many vegetarian dishes (stir-fries, curries, casseroles, chilis, steamed vegetables, salads, and soups, to name a few) are more suited to bowls than to plates. Over the past twelve years, since I changed my diet to a more plant-based diet than before, I have collected a wide variety of both serving bowls and food (eating) bowls for different appetites, serving sizes, food dishes, and aesthetic pleasure. I have gotten most of the bowls cheaply at garage sales and Asian markets.

How much more pleasurable it is to eat from pretty bowls, just the right size for what you want of what you're about to eat!

Sometimes I use a fork, sometimes a spoon. I have a few special spoons that I prefer, with slightly longer, narrower handles and bowls than most teaspoons. If I'm eating a vegetable with no sauce, I prefer a fork.

I also found some small oval plates at an Oriental store, and I use these for omelettes, enchiladas, and other appropriate food. I have mugs for soup and stews.

I rarely eat on a plate. I almost never eat the kind of meal I grew up on, which was meat, potato, vegetable, and salad of some kind. And dessert. And milk. Google milk someday and read what cow's milk does to children. Don't get me started.

Garlic Oil

Use either a whole bulb of garlic, which you will need to peel, or a small bag of fresh already-peeled garlic sometimes available. Place in container, cover with extra virgin olive oil (evoo), and pulse until there are only small bits of garlic visible. Store in container with airtight lid in refrigerator, where it will harden and make a lovely spread.

Use for garlic toast (spread on whole grain bun or bread, and toast in toaster oven so both sides get a little toasty), for garlic bread (cut loaf of whole grain bread, spread on one side of each piece, put back together, wrap in foil, bake in 350° oven until hot and crispy), or when you need just a little for pasta or some other dish.

Peel or Not?

Don't Peel	Peel
Wash well, with a vegetable brush if you have one, or at least under running water. Remove spots and bruises as necessary.	Wash well if done easily, trim ends, then peel. Put peelings in compost. Most of these peels are bitter or tough.

Don't Peel	Peel
Zucchini	Bananas
Summer Squash	Oranges
Potatoes (remove any green spots on skin)	Grapefruit
Tomatoes	Onion
Cucumbers (score with fork before using for easier digestion, or peel if waxy)	Clementines
Carrots	Pineapple
Peppers	Very Large Zucchini
Asparagus	Shallots
Apples	Garlic (smash first)
Asian Pear	Ginger Root & Kiwi (if you don't blend)
Kiwis (if you blend)	Cantaloupe & Watermelon (cut meat from rind)
Berries	Butternut & Acorn Squash (cut meat from rind, or cook first)
Pears, Peaches, Apricots, Plums	

Boiled Dinner

As my assistant Katie would say, *back in the day*, in my La Leche League days I was invited to a St. Patrick's Day party at the home of one of my co-leaders. Both the leaders were of Irish background. As I remember the party was on a weeknight, and the house smelled wonderful when I arrived (my husband was home with the kids). The St. Patrick's Day feast had been simmering all day: a big pot of corned beef, potatoes, cabbage, onions, and carrots. Or at least that is what I remember. Man, was that GOOD. I had a little beer that night, green in color, and several plates of that over-cooked but great smelling, great tasting food.

I have another memory of boiled dinner — the first time I was invited to have dinner at my friend Brice's house, circa 1980. He had me sit at the big oak dining room table in the house he shared with his sister, and he put together a chicken dinner that by my learned rules of cooking should never have worked. The food was *delicious*. He had boiled the chicken with potatoes, onions, carrots, and some other vegetables I wasn't familiar with. *I've caught me a man that cooks,* I thought to myself. Little did I know that he would graduate to curries and stir-fries during our long friendship.

Now in the early spring I like to resurrect those memories by having a boiled dinner of my own. I boil cabbage, potatoes, onions, cauliflower, and carrots, but without the meat! It's not *quite* the same, but good anyway. I can just put it on and when I'm hungry, plate up some food.

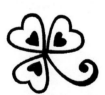  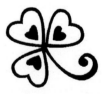

Potatoes O'Brien

Heat a skillet over medium heat and add a thin layer of canola oil. Finely dice potatoes that have been scrubbed but not peeled. Layer in skillet. Turn with a spatula to coat with oil. After about 10 minutes, add diced onion. Turn food and cook for another 10 minutes. Add diced pepper. Turn and cook for another 10 minutes until food is browning and potatoes are tender. Serve with scrambled egg for a high fat, high starch, high protein (high calorie) breakfast.

Irish Potato Bake

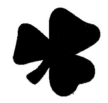

A volume dish you can make ahead. Well worth the effort.

1. Cook in water to cover in a Dutch oven:
   2 lbs potatoes, scrubbed, green & eyes removed, and sliced (don't peel).

2. In a one-quart saucepan over low heat, heat:
   1 1/2 C almond milk
   Add and cook just until tender:
   1 large onion, peeled & chopped
   Set aside, off heat, when done.

3. In a large saucepan cook until tender in water to cover:
   1/2 head green cabbage, quartered, cored, and sliced
   1/2 head napa cabbage (Chinese cabbage), quartered, cored, and sliced
   4 - 6 florets cauliflower

Test potatoes from Step 1 with fork. When tender, drain (save water), dump into a very large mixing bowl, and mash by hand or with an electric mixer.

4. Add onion and almond milk mixture from Step 2 to potatoes, mixing well. Add potato water as needed if mixture is stiff.

5. Mash in cooked, drained cabbages and cauliflower from Step 3 (save water for soup), leaving some small chunks. Add:
   1/4 C extra virgin olive oil
   1/2 t mace (outside of a whole nutmeg, grated)
   2 cloves of garlic, pressed
   sea salt & pepper to taste

Mix well. Spread into flat broiler-proof casserole dishes (like Corning).
Can be refrigerated at this point. (I don't recommend freezing.)

When ready to serve, place under low broiler for 10 minutes or until lightly browned, or heat in 350° oven for 25 - 30 minutes.

Serve family or buffet style, keeping warm on hot tray.

Red Curry Vegetables with Tofu

After Christmas when our bodies need a good cleaning, curry is a great thing to have. This may seem like a formidable list of ingredients, but vegetarian cooks will have most of them on hand as staples.

You'll need:

   1 small jar red curry paste (Thai Kitchen)
   1 12-oz. can light coconut milk
   almond milk (plain, not vanilla)
   fresh basil (can be frozen from last summer's garden)
   vegetable broth
   sweet potato or yam; little red potatoes; carrots
   Vidalia or other sweet onion
   fresh green beans; napa cabbage (Chinese cabbage)
   broccoli or cauliflower; small bok choy or zucchini
   extra firm tofu
   fresh pineapple
   baby spinach; fresh or frozen peas
   garlic; potato flakes

Mix 1 - 3 teaspoons curry paste with one can coconut milk and one cup almond milk in Dutch oven over medium heat. Use 1 teaspoon if you like hot curry, use 2 if you like very hot curry, and 3 if you like spicy hot Thai food. (I use 1 1/2.) Stir frequently until paste is incorporated into milks, then add half a handful of basil, chopped, and some vegetable broth, about 1/2 a cup. Add vegetables and tofu — cleaned, trimmed, cubed, or sliced — as much of each as you want in the order given. Be sure and include some of each.

1/4 to 1/3 block of tofu should be adequate, cut into 3/4" cubes, along with 1 small yam in cubes, 8 little red potatoes halved, 2 large carrots chunked, 1/2 large onion chopped, 10 green beans in 2" pieces, 1/4 napa cabbage, 1/4 cauliflower or 1 stalk broccoli, one small bok choy sliced, 3 thick rings of pineapple cut into chunks, 2 handfuls spinach, 1 C peas, and 4 - 6 cloves garlic, smashed.

Let white and orange vegetables cook some alone before adding green vegetables and tofu. Save spinach, peas, and garlic until the last. If sauce is too thin, add some dried potato flakes or other thickener. Serve with jasmine rice or mixed brown rice.

Orange Almond Stir-fry

I revised this recipe from one my sister Martha found in her local newspaper. It's well worth the extra shopping and cooking: it's better than any dish I've had out at a restaurant. If you're into tofu more than I, use the whole package and cut larger cubes.

Drain on 4 thicknesses of paper towel, pat dry, and cut into 1/2" cubes:
>   **1/2 6-oz package of firm tofu**

Place on platter with marinade made of:
>   **2 T chopped green onion**
>   **2 T tamari sauce**
>   **2 t grated ginger root**
>   **1/2 t olive oil**
>   **2 cloves finely minced garlic**

Toss to coat tofu and let stand for 20 - 30 minutes at room temperature, turning occasionally. Prepare vegetables during this time.

Heat large skillet over medium high heat. Add and swirl around:
>   **2 t canola oil**

Stir fry for 1 minute:
>   **1 baby bok choy,** trimmed and sliced
>   **16 mushrooms,** sliced

Remove tofu from marinade (save) and add to skillet. Stir fry 2 minutes. Add:
>   **1 1/2 C broccoli florets** (about 3 stalks)
>   **1/2 can water chestnuts,** drained, rinsed, and sliced
>   **2 red bell peppers,** thinly sliced

Stir fry for 2 minutes. Add:
>   **2 T tamari sauce**
>   **1 T grated ginger**

Cook, stirring frequently, for 2 minutes or until vegetables are tender but crisp. Add:
>   **20 - 25 snow peas**
>   **reserved marinade**
>   **juice & pulp of 1 orange**

Cook 1 minute, stirring frequently. Remove from heat and serve, topped with:
>   **almond slivers or slices**
>   **sprigs of parsley**

Orange Pecan Stir-Fry

Substitute pecan pieces for the water chestnuts, a small can of mandarin orange segments for the orange, and 1 cup of green peas for the snow peas. Top with pecan halves. Serve either version with cooked brown rice.

Pineapple Fried Rice

I first had pineapple fried rice at the Thai Chili Restaurant in Frenchtown NJ. My version is completely made up from my memory and a sauce recipe my son Dave sent me. Rather than tasting salty like fried rice made with soy sauce or tamari, or yellow and dry like fried rice from a take-out Chinese place, this rice is a bit sweet and full of nutrition. Use leftover white rice the first time if you must, but do try this whole-grain brown or mixed brown rice version.

Heat in deep skillet or wok over medium heat:

1 T olive oil

Prepare and add in the order given, stirring after each addition before preparing next item on list:

1 carrot, diced

1" ginger root, minced

2 T sesame seeds, white, black, or mixed

5 cloves of garlic, smashed and minced

1/2 onion, minced

1 small zucchini, diced but not peeled

1/2 C green peas

2 T apricot preserves

3 T hoisin sauce made with sweet potatoes (like Lee Kum Kee brand)

Stir well and let blend for a few minutes, stirring occasionally. Add:

4 C cooked mixed brown rice

Stir well with spatula or wide wooden spoon, making sure you lift bottom part up and over to further blend.
Add:

1/2 small pineapple, trimmed and chunked
(save some for decoration)

Stir well until all is hot and tasty. Decorate with saved pineapple and additional sesame seeds.

See detailed directions for pineapple prep on page 76.

Yin Yang Fruit

Pick over all fruit for bad spots and stems.

Wash:

    2 C fresh cranberries

Half cover with water; cook with lid on until cranberries "pop." Continue cooking until sauce begins to thicken.

Stir and add:

    1/2 C Sucanat or brown sugar

Stir and add:

    1 C fresh blueberries
    1 C fresh raspberries
    1 C fresh cherries or strawberries, halved

Serve as is or over angel-food cake sliced or cooked rice.

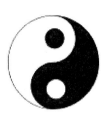

Pad Thai Vegetables

If you have unexpected guests, this stir-fry dish is a fun thing to serve: simple yet elegant, it gets your guests involved in the process of nourishment. Invite your guests to wash their hands and help with the vegetable preparation. What works most smoothly in vegetarian households: one of you does the initial washing and trimming of vegetables, the other cuts them for final use. Guests can also shell peanuts, discarding skins, and crush them in a ziploc bag with a cleaver, stone, or other flat tool.

You'll need:

rice noodles, medium width (1/2 8-oz package)

Bring water just to a boil in a kettle. Cut rice noodles with scissors at points where they fold in the package. Place in a large bowl and pour in hot water to cover. Stir occasionally. When noodles are soft and pliable but *not* mushy (3 - 5 minutes), pour into colander, rinse under cold water, and drain well.

Prepare vegetables as below:

1 medium onion (small dice)

1 carrot (small dice)

1/4 head cauliflower (cut into bite-size pieces)

1 medium zucchini (medium dice)

3 - 4 handfuls baby spinach leaves (washed)

Both these steps can be done ahead of time.

When ready to cook, heat in large skillet over medium-high heat:

1 - 2 T canola oil

Stir fry vegetables in order given above, adding each vegetable to the pan and continuing to stir. I usually use a long-handled hard-plastic spatula for this, folding vegetables in from the outside of skillet to the middle.

Just after adding the spinach, stir in:

drained noodles

2 - 3 T Pad Thai Sauce (< 1/2 8-oz jar Thai Kitchen)

Stir well (a fork-and-spatula technique will help). When well mixed, add:

juice of one lime

Mix well. Add more sauce or some hot water if necessary to make the sauce very light (just coating the vegetables and noodles) and not at all heavy.

Serve in large flat bowls and sprinkle with crushed **raw peanuts.**

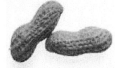

Pad Thai Vegetables 2

1 carrot, scrubbed, trimmed & sliced into rounds
10 green beans, trimmed & cut into 1" pieces
1 onion, peeled, quartered & sliced
1 stalk broccoli, cut into florets
2 - 4 mushrooms, wiped & sliced
1/4 each red, green, yellow, & orange peppers, diced into 3/4" pieces
peanuts

Cook as on opposite page.

Pad Thai Vegetables 3

1 carrot
10 pea pods
10 green beans
1/2 large onion
1 handful soy sprouts
peanuts

Cook as on opposite page.

Pad Thai Vegetables 4

onion
carrot
broccoli
mushrooms
red pepper
spinach
peanuts

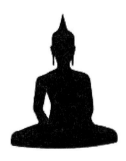

Cook as on opposite page.

Perfect Pork Chops

Apologies to my vegan and Jewish friends who may find this recipe offensive.

Fifty years ago Iowa was and remains now one of the states that produces the most hogs and therefore the most pork. Back when I was a girl, there was nothing better than a hot pork tenderloin sandwich, a pork loin roast with mashed potatoes and gravy, or my mother's pork chops. Now pork is virtually all farmed with the use of antibiotics, pesticides, and other toxins; and hogs are not treated or slaughtered in a very nice way. However, if you get a yen once in a while for meat as I do, find a farmer who uses organic feed for his hogs (I buy from the Amish), and try my mother's braised pork chops. Below that is one of her later pork chop recipes. Mmm . . . delicious!

Purchase two **thick organic pork chops**. Trim any visible fat. Salt and pepper the chops, then sprinkle liberally with flour on both sides.

Over medium heat, heat a skillet with canola oil to cover bottom. Brown the pork chops on one side, then turn with a thin spatula, making sure to get under the coating, and brown other side.

Add **1/2 C water** and put a tight lid on, turning the heat down to low. Simmer for 3/4 hour or until fork tender. Remove to plate and make gravy from the pan drippings: add **2 T flour**, stir with a whisk if you have one, then add **3/4 C almond milk**, stirring until thickened. Add liquid if gravy is too thick. Season as desired. Serve with boiled or mashed potatoes, and a green salad or cooked vegetable.

BBQ Pork Chops

Oven-roast 2 thick organic pork chops in a pan with a lid, using your favorite BBQ sauce on top (I like Open Pit Original). Cook at 300°for two hours, turning frequently. Any pork should be cooked to 190° to kill any resilient critters.

A thought-provoking article on Iowa hog production can be found at: SallyMiller.com/hogs.doc

Pierogi Dinner

Purchase fresh spinach/potato pierogi from your local Amish or Polish market or use frozen pierogi. The Ukrainians make delicious pierogi!

Heat large skillet. Add:
>1 T olive oil

Sauté:
>1/2 large onion, sliced

Add and saute:
>4 regular cultivated mushrooms, sliced

>4 crimini (brown) mushrooms, sliced

Move vegetables to outside of skillet. In middle add and sauté:
>8 spinach/potato pierogi

Turn pierogi once to brown slightly on second side.
Add:
>1/2 to 1 C vegetable broth

Top with:
>4 handfuls baby spinach

Cover skillet until spinach is wilted. Remove cover and stir. Add to taste:
>salt and pepper

Serves 2.

Add an apple salad to round out meal.

Puffs

These light delicious tidbits can be served as an hors d'oeuvre or appetizer. I have included a vegetarian and a tuna version.

Purchase frozen puff pastry (though another day you could make it yourself!). A sheet of puff pastry is approximately 18" x 24" if you can get it from a Thai restaurant, and you will need 1/2 a sheet for each batch of 24. Pepperidge Farm makes a vegan puff pastry with two sheets per package, each of which measures 10" x 10 1/2" and makes about 20.

Tuna Filling:

Mix together:
- **2 small cans of tuna,** rinsed and drained
- **1 clove of shallot,** finely minced
- **1/4 cup peas,** fresh or frozen
- **1 t curry powder**
- **2 T mayo or Miracle Whip**

Vegetarian Filling:

Mix together:
- **1/8 cabbage,** finely minced
- **10 snow peas or green beans,** finely minced
- **1 carrot,** trimmed, scrubbed, and shredded/grated
- **1/2 small onion,** finely chopped
- **1/2 small zucchini,** trimmed, scrubbed, and finely chopped
- **1 t curry powder**
- **1 T mayo or Miracle Whip**

Mix filling well. (I recently mixed mine in a little Cuisinart chopper that came with my Smart Stick immersion blender, pulsing it until it came together, then adding the mayo.) Spread on thawed pastry, having one long edge toward you. Roll up toward the opposite long edge. Wet edge with water and finger seal, then let set, seal side down, preferably in the refrigerator, for at least an hour or two.

Each of these fillings is enough for 20 - 24.

Preheat oven to 400°

Slice roll into slices 1/2" thick and place them on a greased cookie sheet. Put in preheated oven for 20 - 25 minutes or until golden brown. Watch carefully at the end so they don't burn. Loosen puffs just after they come out of the oven and let them cool a bit before serving.

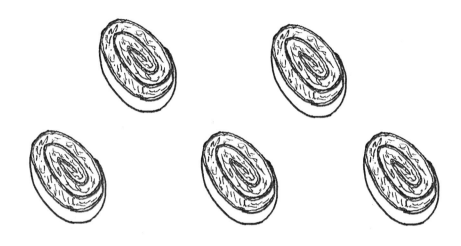

Sauce:

Serve this sauce over the puffs, or place in a bowl — with one of those silver spoons you got from your grandmother or great aunt — and let your guests serve themselves.

Finely dice:
      1 cucumber
      1 red onion
Sprinkle on:
      red hot pepper flakes
Add:
      1/4 C water
      1/4 C vinegar
      2 T sugar
Mix well and chill.

This can also be made in a little chopper.

Frittata

For each person you'll need one egg, beaten with a little water.

In a small skillet over medium low heat sauté in a little olive oil:

1/2 bell pepper, diced

1/2 onion, diced

2 mushrooms, diced

1 stalk broccoli, cut into small pieces of floret

When vegetables are beginning to brown, add egg, making sure it covers bottom of pan. Let egg set for 2 or 3 minutes over a low heat, then lay on top:

1 or 2 slices of pepper jack cheese.

Cover. When cheese is completely melted, serve and enjoy.

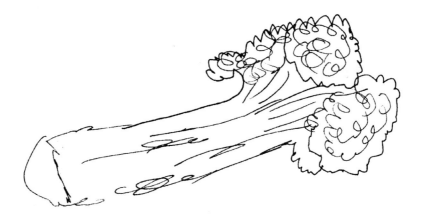

Broccoli with Garlic Sauce

Sometimes after shopping I'm too tired to do anything about food, so on the way home I stop at House of Yeung, my favorite Chinese restaurant and order Broccoli with Garlic Sauce ("Steamed broccoli with garlic sauce on the side"). I take it home and sit down for a few minutes, using the garlic sauce as a dipping sauce for the steamed broccoli. When I feel rejuvenated, I put my groceries away.

Coffee Tea

Years ago I was occasionally troubled with tenderness in my breasts, similar to what a woman feels when her milk is "coming in" in preparation for lactation. Since this was after my childbearing years it was somewhat troubling, and I mentioned it to my then male doctor. He muttered something about how much coffee did I drink, and ordered a baseline mammogram which I have not repeated to this day. I did, however, begin to make coffee with half decaf and half real coffee, so I could continue to drink my nine cups every day.

It was only after my bout with ovarian cancer that I began to read nutritional information and realized how progressive that doctor had been for his time. Indeed, the caffeine in coffee and soda does make lumps and inflammation in your breasts! Lord knows what it does to other parts of the body. If I do go over my line occasionally I get tender breasts, but for the most part I keep a reasonable lid on my caffeine.

I still, however, enjoy the ritual of making coffee and sitting with a cup while I do my email or morning writing. After I got over my love affair with green tea, I looked for a solution. Eventually I hit upon making coffee with regular coffee, but instead of one scoop (2 T) of coffee for each two cups of water, I use one scoop of coffee for every SIX cups of water. This gives me two or three mugs of hot liquid, tasting much like coffee — diner coffee, I'll grant you — with just enough caffeine to help me get going in the morning.

I've made this routine part of my early morning flush. When I first wake up, I drink two or three glasses of water with my morning pills to over-hydrate myself, then the coffee tea helps flush out yesterday's excesses and allows me to start anew. It means a little bit later breakfast, because I allow half an hour between liquids and solid food, and it also means being close to a bathroom. But it all seems to be working well, as I feel better recently than I have in years.

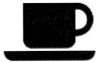

Blood Type A (avoid)

Meat
Seafood
Dairy
Cashews
Kidney, lima, navy beans
Durum wheat
Multigrain bread, pumpernickel
Semolina pasta
Cabbage, mushrooms, tomatoes, green peppers,
 sweet potatoes, yams, black olives
Cantaloupe, bananas, oranges, coconuts
Black pepper, cayenne, vinegar
Ketchup, mayo, pickles, Worcestershire
Beer, liquor, cola, black tea

This is the list of foods I like that are on the avoid list for Blood Type A people, of which I am one. Almost all of these are also things to avoid as a cancer patient or to prevent cancer, with the exception of the alkaline-forming fruits and vegetables: **raw cabbage, mushrooms, tomatoes, green peppers, cantaloupe, bananas, and oranges** — these are all okay in my book, in moderation. Except during early tomato season I wouldn't eat any of the above every day, unless someone brought me Florida oranges fresh off the ground. There is something to say about "fresh," also.

NY Times bestseller *Eat Right 4 Your Type*, where you can find your own list for your blood type, keeps us entirely in the past, and completely ignores the present: our mobile society/world, our intermarriage across cultures, skin color, and body types. Though I keep this list posted on my refrigerator as a reminder, I caution you to use common sense when it comes to food: there is nothing worse than complete denial, which sets up cravings, at least in our minds, if not in our bodies.

Fruit Sorbet Cubes

Originally a Martha Stewart dessert recipe I heard on the run, this vegan version (no animal products) is delicious for breakfast, too!

Rinse 3 empty ice cube trays and chill in freezer.
Blend together:

2 bananas

1 6-oz box fresh raspberries

1/2 C fresh orange juice

1/3 C maple syrup (or to taste)

1 1/2 T fresh lemon or lime juice

Add:

1 C almond milk with vanilla

Blend well and pour into ice-cube trays. Freeze, remove to a large plastic Ziploc bag or container with lid, and store in freezer.

When ready to serve, place 3 - 4 cubes in a small bowl or sherbet dish and serve with a spoon.

Can be re-blended into a slushy if desired, and served in a glass with a straw. Almond Butter Cookies (page 48) make a nice addition to this dessert.

As a variation, use grapes, strawberries, apple, pineapple, pear, blueberries, or other fruit instead of the raspberries. A rainbow of colors makes an especially elegant dessert.

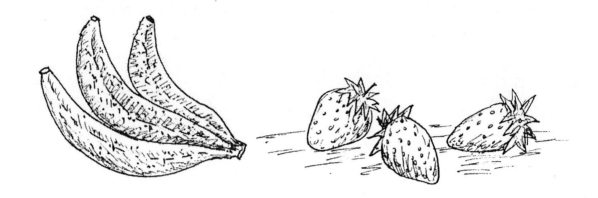

Berry Cherry Bowl

1 **pint ripe strawberries**, rinsed, de-stemmed & cut in half if large
1 **pint blueberries**, rinsed & picked over
2 **C bing cherries**, rinsed & halved, pitted
1/2 **pint raspberries**, rinsed & picked over
2 **ripe bananas**, sliced into thick rounds
2 **T orange or pineapple juice**
1 **t raw sugar** (if necessary for taste)

Prepare fruit and place in a large bowl. Mix gently by using a large spoon, "turning over" the fruit rather then actually stirring, turning the bowl as you're turning the fruit over. Add a little sugar if your body is acidic and the fruit tastes sour. Your body will become more alkaline from eating raw fruits and vegetables.

The juice keeps everything fresh, and the cherries give the berry bowl a little substance. If you won't be serving for several hours, add the banana slices just before serving and mix well.

My assistant Dave M. says you can de-pit the cherries with a heavy-duty straw, then cut in half, or do it the way I learned from my mother: run the tip of a sharp paring knife around the cherry, going all the way to the pit, then twist the two halves apart, digging out the pit with your thumbnail.

Brice's Curry

On days when I've had a long day and don't want to cook dinner, I can often talk Brice into fixing a stir-fry or curry while I continue working. Lucky me!

Put liquids and curry paste in a Dutch oven. Stir well.

      1 pint vegetable broth
      2 cans coconut milk
      3 heaping t red curry paste

When hot, cut up vegetables in order given, adding each to hot liquid, stirring after each addition.

Vegetables, coarse cut:

      3 carrots
      1 medium yam
      2 small Irish potatoes
      1 large onion
      1 1/2 C broccoli
      1 C cauliflower
      1/2 C mushrooms
      1/2 C asparagus
      5 cloves garlic
      1 C red/green/orange peppers

When vegetables are done to your taste (Brice likes them crunchy; I like mine softer), serve over jasmine brown rice (from freezer). Sometimes he thickens it with potato flakes.

Strawberry Shortcake

From Susie Bright

I have at least a 100 witnesses to back me up: this is the best shortcake you've ever tasted. You can go from thinking of it to eating it, in a half-hour flat.

6 C sliced strawberries (3 - 4 little baskets)
1/4 C sugar
2 C flour
2 t baking powder
1 stick cold butter cut into chunks
1 beaten egg
2/3 C milk
Whipped cream

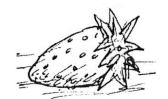

Preheat oven to 450°

Stir the berries and quarter cup of sugar in a bowl, smashing it up a bit with a potato masher. Smush some and leave some intact. Don't over-think it. Set aside.

Get out your Cuisinart and say aloud, "Thank you, god." Now put the dry ingredients into its bowl and pulse them, dry, for a few seconds to mix them up. You have just eliminated the sifting step.

Now cut your cold stick of butter up into chunks (don't over-think that part either) and dump them into the Cuisinart bowl.

Pulse about seven or eight times, one second per pulse. The mixture will look like coarse crumbs. It's supposed to be irregular. That's what makes the flake so tender.

Pour the milk in a measuring cup and then add the egg. Mix them up together.

Now transfer the batter from the Cuisinart into a mixing bowl and add the egg/milk. Stir just enough to moisten it all. *Don't give it a second thought.*

Grease a round cake pan, 8 or 9 inches. Spread the batter in. If you want to get fancy, build up the edge a bit more than the middle. But that's just for looks.

Bake 15 - 20 minutes, or until a toothpick stuck in the center comes out clean. It will be golden on top.

Cool in the pan for 10 minutes. Cut it into slices like it was a cake.

When you lift out a slice for a serving, lay it on your plate and split it into two layers. Spoon the strawberries and whipped cream between the layers and over the top.

If you know you're going to devour the whole thing in one sitting, you could lift the entire cake out of the pan and split it into half to layer it with strawberries and cream. That makes a spectacular sight if you want to make a big entrance.

Since I eat this nearly every hot summer day, I tend to just slice it out a slice at a time, and cut/layer it with strawberries, peaches, mangoes, cherries, whatever — and spray the whipped cream all over.

With the aid of a Cuisinart, this doesn't take five minutes more than you'd spend on a Bisquick recipe. The shortcake is UNREAL BUTTERY GOOD. Once you see the crumb technique, where butter and dry ingredients are lightly handled, you'll understand the secret of making great biscuits, pie crust, etc. Most importantly, you'll never eat one of those turdy hockey-puck shortcakes from the supermarket again.

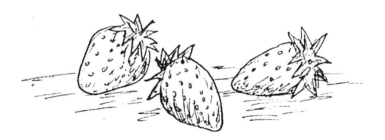

Strawberries and Cream

When I read this delicious-sounding recipe on Susie Bright's blog I thought to myself, *there must be a way to have this taste, but in a healthier way!* Besides, I had no Cuisinart.

I figured out how to sugar the strawberries just a little with raw sugar and just before serving add a dollop of coconut cream, the fat part of coconut milk, which you can scoop off the top of a regular can of coconut milk that has been chilled (I keep a can in the refrigerator during strawberry season). I have served this several times, and my guests all like the natural flavor of the coconut cream over the down side of cow's cream or manufactured cream. None of us even missed the shortcake, and the white cream satisfied our visual desires for whipped cream.

Strawberry Dip

Easy and delicious. Can be used as an appetizer, dessert or aphrodisiac. Perfect in May when the strawberries come out.

Break organic chocolate bar into ceramic or glass ramekin (1/2 bar/person). Place ramekin over hot water in saucepan over medium/low heat.

Prepare strawberries by washing well. Remove bad spots with a small paring knife but leave stems for easier handling.

When chocolate is melted, remove ramekin to plate and surround with strawberries. Serves to 2 - 3 people. Melt additional chocolate in a second ramekin while enjoying the first with your guests.

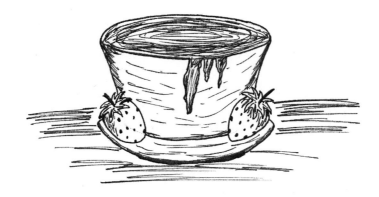

Fruit and Vegetable Washes

Water, especially running water, is necessary and sufficient for washing fruits and vegetables. I suggest a special brush that you keep just for vegetables; most fruits are too delicate to use a brush on. Please stay away from "washes" that are sold in grocery stores. They contain material toxic to the human body. Why bother and expend the money? Don't be taken in by every ad you see.

As you eat more fruits and vegetables, especially organic ones, your body will begin to cleanse itself. Eventually you will be able to taste "washes" that are used on lettuce and other salad ingredients in restaurants. Ask to have some "unwashed" or rinsed under water only.

Fruit Rolls

Substitute for a sweet roll at breakfast, or serve as a dessert after a light soup and salad dinner. Scrumptious! Can be rolled ahead of time and held in refrigerator until cooking time. Plan to serve soon after cooking, as they do not save well.

Thaw 8" egg roll wrappers or puff pastry (usually purchased frozen). Remove 2 - 3 per person you are going to serve and refreeze the rest, well wrapped. Place a small flat dish of water near your workspace.

For each 6 - 7 rolls, slice:

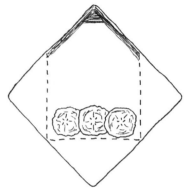

> **1 ripe banana**

Wash and pick over:

> **1/2 C cranberries** (fresh or frozen)

Core and cut up into small chunks:

> **2 slices fresh pineapple**

Assemble rolls by placing a wrapper in front of you on your workspace at an angle, a corner toward you. Off center place horizontally:

> **3 slices banana**

On top of banana slices place:

> **5 cranberries**
>
> **6 - 8 small chunks pineapple**

Roll up as an egg roll, front corner over fruit, sides folded over towards middle, then roll up fairly tightly. When you get to where it looks like a bulging fat envelope, stick your finger (clean, of course) into the little bowl of water and wet the edges of the triangle still showing (where the glue might be on an envelope), and across where the fruit ends. Then roll snuggly up to the point and place point-side down on a doubled piece of paper towel. Let set up until ready to sauté, but at least ten minutes. If the last roll has an odd number of fruit pieces or if it looks skimpy, add a small piece of:

> **chocolate candy** (kisses, drops, or bars)

For dessert you may put chocolate in every third or fourth roll for a surprise!

Heat skillet over medium heat and add thin layer of canola oil. Turn temperature down a bit and sauté rolls on both sides until golden brown, adding oil as necessary. Drain and cool on paper towel. Transfer to serving plate and let guests help themselves. Make sure you supply ample paper napkins.

Apples, raspberries, blueberries, peaches, or other ripe fruit can be used, but keep the banana in. With ripe (sweet) banana, the cranberries provide a tiny burst of sour, and are the best berry to use. For those stuck on toppings, serve a bowl of "white stuff" — coconut cream, whipped cream, non-dairy topping, yogurt, soy yogurt, or sour cream.

Vegetable Spring Rolls

Combine ingredients all finely chopped or shredded:

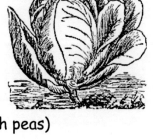

- **1 small zucchini squash**, shredded
- **8 - 10 baby spinach leaves**, chopped
- **1 C napa cabbage** (1/4 head), chopped
- **1 C cabbage** (1/4 head), chopped
- **8 - 10 green beans**, chopped (asparagus or fresh peas)
- **8 - 10 pea pods**, chopped
- **1 carrot**, shredded
- **4 - 5 scallions** or purple onion, chopped
- **5 regular mushrooms**, chopped
- **1" ginger**, grated

This is similar to Oriental dumplings. Use egg roll wrappers, and see the fruit roll recipe on page 117 for rolling technique.

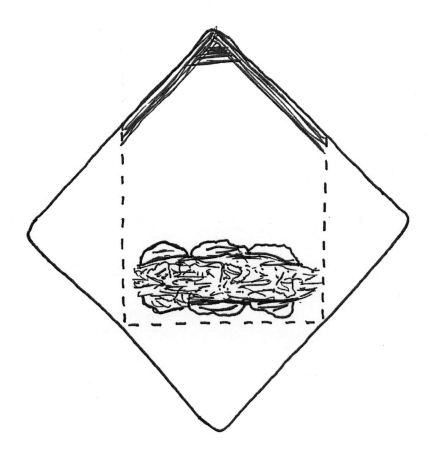

Vegetable Broth

Blended Broth

My vegetable broth is very nutritious and easy to make. The idea is to infuse the water with nutrients without killing them all off from too high a heat. The night before you shop, take all your old vegetables (those you haven't used for a stir-fry or a curry), scrub well, and cut into chunks. In a Dutch oven or other suitable pan place vegetables along with any uneaten garden salad, cover with water and any vegetable water you have saved in the freezer, bring to a simmer, reduce heat, and let cook slowly until vegetables are tender. Use a blender or immersion blender to blend all the vegetables and water. Cool. Package in pint-size Chinese soup containers, cap, label, and freeze for future use.

Concentrated Broth

When you have the time, after blending, let the broth cook down over low heat until half to two thirds the volume. Cool, package, and mark. Takes up less room in the freezer.

Clear Broth

Strain broth before or after blending. The blended and strained broth will be less clear but more nutritious. Use the strained-only broth for hot and sour soups or light-colored soups such as potato or cauliflower. Blended broth is usually green.

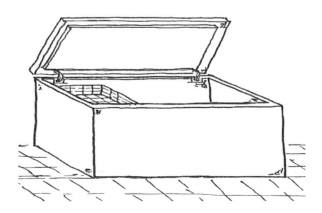

Protein in Plant Foods

Here are the percentages of protein by calories in some plant foods. We all need ≈ 10% of our calories from protein, so it's obvious that with a variety of fruits and vegetables this goal is easily attainable.

soybean sprouts	54% protein
spinach	49% protein
broccoli	45% protein
kale	45% protein
Mung bean sprouts	43% protein
cauliflower	40% protein
bamboo shoots	39% protein
mushrooms	38% protein
Chinese cabbage	34% protein
lettuce	34% protein
green peas	30% protein
lentils	29% protein
zucchini	28% protein
navy, kidney, lima beans	26% protein
cucumbers	24% protein
cabbage	22% protein
pumpkin seeds	21% protein
tomatoes, peanuts	18% protein
whole wheat	17% protein
lemons, onions	16% protein
oatmeal, beets	15% protein
walnuts, sesame seeds	13% protein
almonds, cashews	12% protein
barley, potatoes	11% protein
pecans	10% protein
honeydew melon	10% protein
brown rice, yams	8% protein
watermelon, oranges	8% protein
strawberries, cherries	8% protein
grapes, filberts	8% protein

Source: *Nutritive Value of American Foods in Common Units, USDA Handbook No. 45*

Cinco de Mayo Salad

This recipe came from my sister, culled from the Minneapolis Star Tribune. *I like this version so much better than most black bean salads because it uses rice instead of corn. Sometimes I buy the colored peppers already cut into strips and just dice them into the salad. All the colors make it look very festive! A great salad to take to a picnic in the summer, too!*

Thaw, rinse, and drain:
> 2 C cooked black beans

Thaw and put into a large bowl:
> 2 C cooked mixed brown rice

Add:

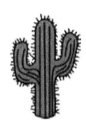

> 1 yellow pepper, diced
> 1 green pepper, diced
> 1 C diced celery
> 3-4 scallions, chopped (use white and some green)
> 1 handful cilantro leaves, chopped

Add the drained black beans and mix.

In a large Pyrex cup put:
> 1/2 C mild salsa
> 1/2 C Wishbone Italian dressing
> juice of 1 lime
> 1 t ground cumin

Whirl with immersion blender. Pour half of dressing over salad (save rest for another time) and mix well. Serve at once or refrigerate until needed, up to 4 days. Stir every once in a while to keep flavors blending well. Top with sliced ripe plum tomatoes just before serving.

Enchiladas

Make a double recipe of salad above. Use half for delicious easy enchiladas. Use any kind of tortilla or wrap, large ones preferred. Place heaping rectangle of salad across middle of wrap. Sprinkle with shredded cheddar, mozzarella, or pepper jack cheese. Roll up and place in casserole dish or ovenproof plate. Top with slices of pepper jack cheese. Heat in 350° oven for 20 - 25 minutes or until cheese is melted and enchilada is hot.

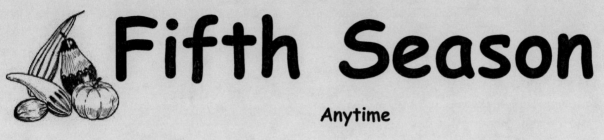

Fifth Season

Anytime

Fifth Season Contents (continued)

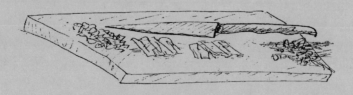

4-Bean Chili Starter

Soak overnight:
>1 lb dried soybeans

In a separate bowl, soak overnight:
>1 lb dried kidney beans
>1 lb dried adzuki beans

In morning heat on stovetop until hot:
>8 pts water/broth combination

Rinse and add soybeans. Cook for one hour over low heat. (Soybeans take an extra hour so need to be started first.)

Rinse second bowl of beans and add to pot. When beans are hot, add:
>1 C green, yellow, red, or a mixture of split peas

The split peas are added to thicken chili. Cook for 2 hours. Add room-temperature water as needed to keep beans covered.

Add **onion, carrot, and celery,** about 2 cups each. Cook an hour. At this point chili can be frozen for later use. Spices don't freeze well, so add spices later.

When you are ready to finish the chili, thaw several quarts of starter and heat over stovetop. Add in order given, stirring after each addition:
>**2 pints tomato sauce,** thawed (or 1 large can tomato sauce)
>**ground red pepper** (start with half a teaspoon, adding more to taste)
>**chili powder** (start with a tablespoon, adding more to taste)

>**cauliflower,** chopped
>**green beans,** chopped
>**corn**
>**peas**

Add as much as you have of the vegetables or as much as you want/like, but at least two cups of each vegetable. Cook until vegetables are tender and sauce is thick and succulent.

Serve in large bowls or over cornbread (p.34).
See page 33 for another version of this, starting with cooked beans.

Last Stew of Summer

To use up the last of the tomatoes and zucchini, remove stem and any bad spots from a large bag of:

tomatoes

Cut into rough dice and heat in a large soup pot or Dutch oven on medium-low. When tomatoes begin to look like chunky sauce, add:

6 - 8 C cooked kidney beans from freezer (see page 29 for method)

1/2 stalk celery, sliced across all ribs

4 carrots, sliced

1 large onion, diced

When vegetables are tender, add:

1 large can tomato purée

1 large zucchini, diced with skin left on, but some of seeds removed

Cook until squash is tender, stirring often. Add pepper or other seasoning.

Bean Food

Soak 8 hours:

2 lbs pinto beans (≈ 5 C dried)

1 lb black-eyed peas (≈ 2 1/2 C)

Heat over stovetop in a large soup pot or Dutch oven until hot:

1 gal water (8 pints)

4 pts vegetable broth

Rinse soaked beans well under running water. Add to broth mixture. Also add:

1/2 lb dried red lentils

Cook for 2 hours, stirring often on stovetop, or cook in 250°oven, stirring every half hour. After 2 hours, add and cook on medium-low until tender:

1/2 celery stalk (cut across whole stalk)

4 carrots, chopped

Then add in order given and cook until tender, stirring frequently:

4 regular potatoes, diced small

2 leeks, chopped

8 kale leaves, chopped

1/4 green cabbage, chopped

Package for the freezer what you don't eat. Though plain, you'll love it in the winter and early spring when you don't feel like cooking. Heat a pint in a small saucepan to have with rice or noodles. Add other vegetables as desired.

Concert Chili

Soak overnight or for 8 hours:

    2 C red kidney beans

    2 C Anastasia beans

    2 C cranberry beans

Rinse and place in a large soup pot. Add:

    8 pts broth/water

Heat on stovetop until hot. Put in 250° oven for 2 hours.
Add:

    3 pts tomato sauce or **chunks**

    2 C celery (1/2 stalk), diced

    2 C carrots, sliced

    2 C onion (1 large), diced

Bake in the oven for 1 - 2 hours, then add:

    2 small zucchini, diced

    1/2 head cauliflower, florets

    1 - 2 T chili powder

Add last:

    1 green pepper, diced

    1 red pepper, diced

    1 yellow/orange pepper, diced

Stir and cook until done to your liking. Serve in bowls with a little cheddar cheese grated on top, or a dollop of sour cream. Add more spice if you like it hotter.

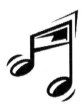 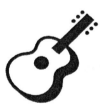

Chili Mac

Make some macaroni. Layer it with any of the chilis in this book and shredded cheese — cheddar and a little mozzarella. Top with shredded pepper jack or cheddar cheese. Heat in a 350° oven for 25 to 30 minutes, or until hot and bubbly. See page 35 for a more detailed description (though don't add the milk!).

Fall Bean Stew

Soak (each in separate bowls):
   1 lb soybeans
   1 lb pinto beans (3 3/4 C)
Rinse soybeans well and place in a large soup pot or Dutch oven. Add:
   1 gallon water (8 pints)
Cook soy beans for 1 hour, add the other beans and
   4 pints vegetable broth

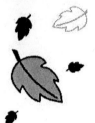

Stir well and add:
   1/2 lb green split peas
Cook over low heat for 2 hours. Add:
   4 carrots, quartered lengthwise & sliced across
   2 - 3 medium yellow onions (use half now, save half for crunch later)
   1/2 celery stalk, sliced across all ribs
Cook for 1 hour, stirring occasionally. Add:
   1 head cauliflower, separated into florets, cut if too large for a bite
Cook for 1/2 hour.
Wash well and chop:
   5 - 7 leaves of kale
   5 - 7 leaves of Swiss chard
Add to stew and stir. Add:
   2 medium green or yellow squash, cut into 1/4" slices, plus saved onions
Cook until tender, approximately 10 - 15 minutes.
Serve and enjoy.

Freeze leftovers for future suppers when you're deep in the middle of a project and don't want to stop to cook.

Plain Beans

Rinse 3 cups pinto, kidney, or other beans. Soak all day. Rinse well. Cook overnight on low in crockpot. Turn up in morning, adding water as necessary. Cook until tender. Makes 4 + pints.

International Bean Stew

Soak:

    1 C dried soybeans (in separate bowl)

    2 C pinto beans

    1 C kidney beans

After 8 hours or more, rinse soybeans well and place in a large soup pot or large Dutch oven. Cover with:

    4 C water

Cook for one hour. Add:

    4 C concentrated vegetable broth

Rinse pinto and kidney beans. Add to pot, and add additional water to cover by 1". Cook for 1 hour. Then add:

    1/2 C mung beans

    1/2 C French lentils

    1/2 C red lentils (or split green peas)

Bring almost to a boil, then turn heat down to low and add:

    2 leeks, chopped

    2 carrots, chopped

    1/4 celery stalk, chopped across all ribs and leaves

Cook for 1 hour, then add:

    1 small bok choy, chopped

    1/2 cauliflower, divided into florets

Stir every 10 minutes for about 1/2 hour.

Poison

dry mouth	drowsiness
nausea	headache
vomiting	muscle pain
diarrhea	constipation

These are the "side effects" of pharmaceutical drugs you hear about on TV and see in magazines. They are also ways your body has of telling you that you've just been poisoned and you need to drink more water to help flush your blood from the toxin. Yes, if you keep taking the drug you will eventually get used to it, but that doesn't deny the toxicity. It's better to stay with natural remedies if and when you can.

Cranberry Oatmeal Dessert

Preheat oven to 350°

Melt in oven in a 10" x 15" baking pan:

    1/2 C margarine or butter

Add:

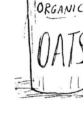

    2 C cranberries, washed and picked over

    1 C Sucanat

Stir until well mixed and return to oven until berries are slightly softened, 5 - 10 minutes. Mash down with back of spatula. Stir in:

    2 mashed bananas (mash on a flat dish or plate)

    2 C oatmeal

In the meantime, place in a large mixing bowl:

    1 white cake mix

    2 eggs

    1 1/4 C juice (orange, pineapple, or other)

    1 C cranberries, washed and picked over

    1 C nuts, broken into pieces

Mix well by hand. Spoon out cake batter onto top of prepared fruit in pan.

Bake for 40 - 45 minutes or until golden brown.

See page 77 for removal method (upside down on large tray). Serves 20 - 24.

Sweet Puffs

Use frozen puff pastry. Thaw as instructed and roll out on a lightly floured board. Spread a sweet filling, such as chopped mincemeat, fruit preserves, poppy seed filling, or butter/sugar/cinnamon/maple syrup. Roll up, seal edge, and let sit in refrigerator for at least an hour, covered.

Preheat oven to 350°

Slice the pastry into 1/4" spirals. Place on a greased cookie sheet. Bake at 350° for 20 to 25 minutes, or until golden brown. Makes 24 - 30.

Serve with fruit.

Molasses Cookies

Preheat oven to 350°

Mix:
      1/2 C Grade B maple syrup
      1/2 C molasses
      1/4 C brown sugar
      1/4 C sesame oil
      1/4 C applesauce or 1 small mashed banana

Sift together in a large bowl:
      1 1/2 C whole wheat flour
      1/2 C other flour
      2 T ground ginger
      1 1/2 t baking powder
      1/2 t ground cinnamon
      1/4 t ground cloves
      1/4 t baking soda
Add:
      1/2" peeled ginger root, finely grated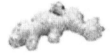

Add liquids and mix.

Mix together:
      1/2 t vinegar
      1 T water
Add this mixture to dough and mix well.

Let dough sit for 5 minutes.

Drop by teaspoonfuls onto greased cookie sheet and bake in preheated oven for 10 minutes. Don't let them burn!

Serve with fruit or berries. Makes 24 medium cookies.

Salmon Casino

Preheat oven 350°

In a large bowl, mix:

> 1 **small egg**, slightly beaten
> 1/4 **C hemp milk**
> 1/4 **C whole wheat bread crumbs**
> 1 **T butter**, melted
> 1 **T onion**, finely chopped
> 1 **T lime juice**
> **salt & pepper** (as desired at end)

Mix in:

> 1 **large can (15-oz) salmon**, drained, skeleton removed, and meat flaked
> with a fork

Place a wax paper lining in a 3″ x 7″ loaf pan and add salmon mixture.

Bake at 350° for 30 - 40 minutes or until brown. Remove from oven and take off wax paper right away or it will stick. If you like it crisper, return to oven for 5 to 10 minutes.

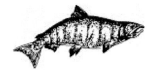

Serve with sauce below.

Lime Butter Sauce

In a small pitcher heat for 15 seconds in the microwave or until melted:

> 2 **T butter**

Add:

> 1 **T fresh parsley**, finely chopped
> 1 **T fresh or frozen chives**, finely chopped
> 1/8 **t dried tarragon**, crumbled

Microwave for 10 seconds. Then add:

> **juice of 1 lime**

Serve over Salmon Casino, above. Can be kept warm over a votive candle.

This was a favorite of my family when the kids were growing up. For me it was reminiscent of the salmon loaf and salmon croquettes my mother used to make.

Meatloaf

My mother used to make a meatloaf with 2 pounds pork and 1 pound veal. Over the years I have switched entirely to beef for meat loaf, which I find comforting about 6 times a year.

These are my ingredients, which I never measure, so it is a bit different every time. I got the idea of using beef from Sue, my older sister *(everybody uses ground beef)*. The vegetables, which I thought of, help with the digestion process, as meat has no fiber.

> **1/2 lb ground chuck & 1/2 lb ground round**
> **egg, soy or almond milk** (about 3/4 C), **whole grain bread crumbs, onion, ketchup, mushrooms, shredded carrots, maybe some chopped spinach, salt, garlic, and a bit of vegan Worcestershire sauce.** Occasionally I add **peas** for color, or chopped **green beans.**

Mix well and bake at 350° for an hour, or 400° for 45 minutes or until browned.

Hamburger Pie

This is a favorite of my daughter Chris from her growing-up days.

Make your favorite meatloaf recipe and spread in a large pie plate, making sure it goes up the sides. Bake for a little less time than usual (because of its thinness). Remove from oven and drain any fat off. Around the edges pipe or drop spoonfuls of mashed potatoes (try them with the skins left on). Fill the middle with cooked peas. Sprinkle shredded cheddar cheese over the potatoes. All of this can be done ahead of time.

When ready to serve, place under broiler for a few minutes until cheese melts, or warm in the microwave if you have used a Pyrex pie pan. Cut into wedges. Children love this.

Chicken Salad

In large bowl mix together:
> **1 chicken breast**, cooked & diced
> **1/2 C celery**, cut across whole stalk about 5 times
> **1/2 C pecans**, broken into small pieces
> **1/4 onion**, finely diced
> **extra virgin olive oil**
> **lime zest**
> **juice of 1 lime**

Summer Menu

Zen Iced Tea (p.133)

Steamed Asparagus, Cauliflower, Broccoli

Fruity Salad (p.133)

Moving Day Menus

1st Day: Lasagna or Chili Mac (p.125)
Green Garden Salad (p.21)

2nd Day: Chicken Salad (p.131)
Mediterranean Potato Salad (p.4)
Cinco de Mayo Salad (p.121)

3rd Day: Vegetable Pizza (p.57)
Green Garden Salad (p.21)

Dessert all days: Watermelon
&
Cantaloupe
both cut in wedges
for eating by hand

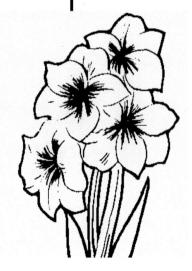

Zen Iced Tea

4 Zen tea bags (made by Tazo)
5 to 5 1/2 C water

In large teakettle boil water, remove from heat, and steep tea bags in a teapot.
Remove tea bags after 3 - 4 minutes.
Let tea cool some. Fill a large pitcher 1/4 full of water. Add tea.
Fill individual tall glasses with a sprig of mint & ice cubes, pour tea over, and enjoy!

Fruity Salad

Mix together in a large bowl:
  3 - 4 clementines, peeled and separated into pieces
  2 apples, diced small
  1 Asian pear, diced small (big like an apple, crisp, but tastes like a pear)
  1/2 pt blueberries
  1/2 C dried cranberries
  pineapple, chunks, a good amount
  grapes, a good amount

Pour **orange juice** over and mix. Chill and serve.
This makes a larger salad than the one below.

Fruity Salad 2

Mix together in large bowl:
  1/2 C dried cranberries
  1 rib of celery, diced
  1 carrot, shredded
  1 ripe banana, sliced
  navel orange, peeled and separated into pieces
  strawberries, sliced

Pour orange or pineapple juice over and mix. Chill and serve.

One-Pan Pasta

Prepare vegetables while bringing water to a boil for pasta and broccoli: (see page 73 for method)

1 C Amish "dumplings" or other pasta like bows or Campanelle
1 stalk broccoli, cut into florets

2 t extra virgin oil (evoo)
1/4 Vidalia onion, diced
1/2 red pepper, diced
1 handful of pea pods, chopped
Parmigiano-Reggiano cheese, grated

Save the Gravy

Gravy, Chili, Stew & Beans 1st Aid

If you get a phone call or another distraction, and your pot of gravy, chili, stew, or beans seems to have stuck on the bottom, *resist the impulse to stir it vigorously!* First, remove the pot from the heat. Don't turn the fire off, but physically remove the pot to another burner that is not on. Let it sit a minute or two. *Gently* stir it, starting at the edges of the pot. Do the upper 7/8ths, avoiding the stuck part on the bottom middle. Let the pan sit off heat for 5 to 10 minutes, then begin to stir gently again, starting with the outside circle and gradually going into the center. I have found that with this method, my gravy, chili, stew, or beans come up from the bottom quite nicely if I'm just patient.

If it is *burned* smelling, remove from stove, let cool, and ladle the top half to 2/3 into another pot to finish cooking, being careful to stir frequently. Adding a bit of water will help.

Leftover-Rice Lunch

Heat in large skillet/wok over medium heat:
>   **1 t canola oil**

Sauté:
>   **1/2 onion**, diced

Add and stir:
>   **1 C peas**
>   **1/3 - 1/2 C pecans**, broken into pieces

Add and heat:
>   **1 1/2 C cooked brown rice**

Season to taste with:
>   **1 - 3 t tamari sauce** (low sodium)

The food aisles are nothing more than one large carbohydrate divided up into different packages, all of them beckoning you to take them home and gobble them up. — Barry Sears

---

Leftover-Rice Lunch 2

Heat in large skillet/wok over medium heat:
>   **2 t canola**

Add and stir-fry:
>   **8 green beans**, chopped
>   **1/2 medium zucchini**, diced
>   **1 stalk broccoli**, florets
>   **1 handful baby spinach**, chopped
>   **1 plum tomato**, diced

Stir and let cook a bit.

Then turn heat to low, add and mix in:
>   **1 1/2 C cooked mixed brown rice**

Put lid on to heat thoroughly (like a sweat lodge). Stir and enjoy.

Striped Macaroni

I first had this at the home of a young English woman. Our husbands had both just started to work at IBM in Westchester County, NY and we became good friends — even staying up all night playing "English Monopoly" during a blizzard. Hazel served this in stripes across a large platter, and what a pretty sight it was — reds, green, white — with a gravy boat full of the cheesy sauce. Each guest could take what s/he wanted.

During my children's growing up years I used to struggle to make this and have it all come out hot, delicious, and attractive. All those pots to wash afterwards (this was before dishwashers) and leftovers to deal with.

Suddenly one year I thought, *I'll just make a casserole out of this. Should taste the same!* It did. I can now make this — using some of that leftover Christmas or Easter ham — in the morning, when my energy level is higher, and heat it up whenever it is wanted.

It makes a wonderful casserole. You still have the same number of pans to wash, but you can get them done up early in the day or the day before. Use whatever amounts of ingredients that you wish.

1. Cooked **elbow macaroni**
2. **Ham strips** - 1/3" x 1/3" x 2 1/2" long, sautéed in canola oil with dried oregano crumbled in
3. Slices of **tomatoes** sautéed in **butter** and **basil** (in a pinch I've used whole canned tomatoes)
4. Cooked **green peas**
5. Cheese sauce (cream sauce p.137 with shredded **cheddar cheese** added)

If they get done at different times, just let them sit and cool until all are ready to be assembled.

Make it like any casserole — layer the macaroni first, then some ham, then some peas, tomatoes, and cover with sauce. Repeat layers.

Bake covered at 350° for 25 - 30 minutes or until hot and bubbly. Remove lid for the last ten minutes.

Au Gratin Potatoes

Preheat oven to 400°

Prepare:
> **2 medium red-skinned potatoes**, scrubbed, de-eyed, quartered, and sliced into 1/4" slices
> **2 medium brown-skinned potatoes**, as above
> **1 red onion**, diced

Layer potatoes, onions, and **1/2 C shredded cheese** in a 9" x 9" casserole dish.

In a sauce pan over medium-low heat place:
> **1 T olive oil**
> **1 T whole grain flour**

Stir and cook until bubbly. Slowly add:
> **1 C plain soy milk**

Cook until it begins to thicken. Add another **1/2 C shredded cheese**. Pour sauce over potatoes and place in preheated oven. Cook until tender and brownish on top, approximately 45 to 50 minutes. For a "juicier" dish, double ingredients for sauce. Let sit for 5 - 10 minutes (can add more time if needed) before serving.

Cauliflower Au Gratin

To make cream sauce mix together:
> **2 T extra virgin olive oil**
> **2 T flour**

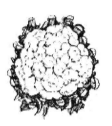

Cook and stir until bubbly. Add:
> **1 C almond or hemp milk**
> **1 C shredded cheddar cheese**

Meanwhile, par-boil or lightly steam:
> **1 head of cauliflower**, broken up into florets

Add to casserole dish, pour sauce mixture over cauliflower. Bake in 350° oven for 30 minutes. Add to top:
> **bread crumbs (p.18)**

Bake until brown and bubbly, 5 - 10 minutes.

Salad Rap

After a busy Monday I often collapse in front of the TV at 8 PM, exhausted, hungry, with no maid in sight! A salad wrap is easy to fix, easy to digest and not too heavy for late eating. Here is where a ready-made salad is indispensable — bite size greens and vegetables, not huge lumps of raw food. What you might put before a queen who wants to maintain her dignity, not chomp and tear at her food like an uncivilized caveman.

Train a helper to make a good salad, when you can, this helps. Husband, boy-friend, child. Help a relative, aunt, or friend with salads. Do salads together or pay someone to do it for you. See suggestions on page 21.

Carrot Spinach Salad

Wash, towel dry, and stack **10 - 12 large leaves of spinach**. With large knife slice into very thin strips. Turn stack and cut strips into 1" pieces. Rinse, drain, and add to medium-size bowl.

Grate **2 small carrots** into bowl.

Add any dressing; mix and eat.

Cabbage Tuna Salad

1/4 head of green cabbage, cut into thirds and sliced thin
1 small can tuna, drained
1/6 stalk of celery, sliced thin across all ribs
1 small onion, minced fine
1 - 2 T mayo (I use Miracle Whip)
1/4 - 1/2 C leftover rice (optional)

Mix well and chill before eating.

Summer Sandwich

cracked wheat or other whole grain roll
salad dressing, as desired
lettuce, paring center rib so lettuce leaf is more pliable
cukes, Kirby, sliced
tomatoes, sliced
mint leaves
baby spinach

Arrange mint and spinach on roll, add other ingredients, with lettuce and top of roll on top.

Quick Bruschetta

basil
oregano
olive oil
tomatoes
peppers
onions

Mix together and let sit for 1/2 hour.

In the meantime, cut whole wheat bread (long loaf) into slices, spray with extra virgin olive oil. Broil until toasted.

When ready to serve, round vegetables on top of toast.

Fall Breakfast Drink

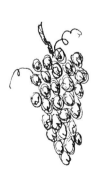

1 banana
1 bunch of any kind of grapes red, Concord or
      champagne (I remember Concord from our
      Victory Garden during World War II)
Blend until smooth and drink.

Onion Soup

Sauté over low heat in butter or evoo until soft:

    2 Vidalia onions, peeled, halved, then sliced thin

Add:

    3 C vegetable broth
    salt and pepper

Let simmer 20 - 30 minutes.

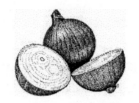

Meanwhile toast **rolls** or **whole grain bread**, sliced thick, on both sides.

When ready to serve ladle soup into oven proof bowls, top with toast and shredded **mozzarella cheese**.

Place under broiler until cheese melts. Serve with **grated parmesan cheese** on top.

Vegetable Pea Soup

Cook covered over low heat for 1/2 hour:

    10 C water
    2 C dried split peas or **1 C green**, **1 C yellow dried split peas**
    2 onions, chopped
    2 whole bay leaves (remove before serving)

Add:

    2 carrots, chopped
    2 potatoes, chopped
    1 C celery, chopped
    4 T parsley
    1 T basil, chopped (or 1 t dried basil, crumbled)
    1 t dried thyme

Cook another half hour or until vegetables are tender.

Serves 6

Butternut Squash Soup

Preheat oven to 375°

Scrub and place on oven racks:
>   1 large or 2 small butternut squash

Cook for 1/2 hour or until tender when stabbed with a fork. Cool.

Meanwhile, heat in a large soup pot or large Dutch oven over low heat on stovetop:
>   1 qt vegetable broth
>   1 qt water

Add squash meat to broth mixture then add:
>   1 T molasses
>   1 T raw sugar
>   2 t cinnamon
>   1 t cumin, nutmeg, and ginger

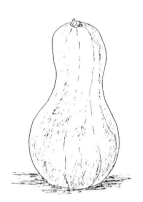

Blend until smooth. Add:
>   1 can coconut milk

Serve with freshly grated nutmeg. Freeze leftovers.

Cabbage Soup

Heat to almost a boil:
>   5 C vegetable broth
>   9 C water

Add:
>   1/2 head of cabbage, sliced
>   3 carrots, sliced
>   1/2 celery stalk, sliced across all ribs
>   5 small potatoes, diced
>   1/2 onion, diced

Cook until vegetables are tender. Add:
>   1 C spinach leaves
>   sea salt (to taste)
>   spices (to taste)

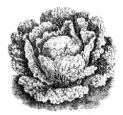

Serve and enjoy. Freeze leftovers.

Green Bean Chowder

In large soup pot over medium heat, add and bring almost to a boil:

- **2 concentrated vegetable broth** (3 C regular broth)
- **6 C water**

Add:

- **1/2 onion**, diced
- **1/2 C celery**, diced
- **4 potatoes**, diced
- **1/4 head of cauliflower**, florets
- **1 small carrot**, diced
- **2 handfuls of green beans** (about 1/2 lb), washed and cut into 1 1/2" lengths
- **cilantro** (optional)
- **1 t sea salt**

Cook until vegetables are tender.

Remove 4 cups of soup to blender and blend, or pulse an immersion blender, leaving some chunks. Simmer until delicious; adjust seasoning as needed.

Christmas Soup

Great Northern beans, **black-eyed peas**, and **lentils** form the base of this delicious thick soup with **carrots**, **celery**, **onions** and **ham bits**. Use nutritious **vegetable broth** as the base.

Pizza Sauce

Heat in Dutch oven over medium heat:
> **1 T organic extra virgin olive oil**

Sauté:
> **6 cloves garlic**, sliced

Stir and add:
> **1 large onion**, chopped

Stir and sauté until onions are soft.

Add tomatoes a few at a time. Never add more than you can easily stir. I found this to be 1" down from the top edge of the Dutch oven. Use:
> **2 - 3 kinds tomatoes** (plum, beefsteak, cherry, etc.) 10 lbs or so, a half-full brown grocery sack, washed, cored, trimmed and diced.

Continue to add diced tomatoes. I use a large bowl to put these in, transferring into Dutch oven when bowl is full.

Cook until tomatoes are softened and reduced. 1" down from the edge of the pot allows ample room for frequent stirring. Cook until thick. Near end add:
> **fresh basil**, chopped
> **fresh oregano**, chopped
> **more garlic**, chopped

This sauce is full of fiber and flavor, well worth the effort.

To make pizza see page 57 for method.

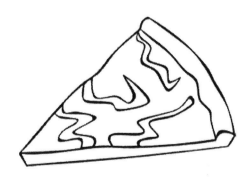

Polynesian Sauce

This wonderful sauce for stir-fries or steamed vegetables comes from the Veggie Works Vegan Cookbook, the project of the former chef at Veggie Works in Belmar, New Jersey, a favorite restaurant down the shore.

Blend until smooth:

     1 1/4" slice fresh pineapple, trimmed & cored

     1/2 C water

     3 slices ginger, peeled

     2 cloves of garlic

Add pineapple juice to make 2 cups. Place in saucepan over low heat. Add:

     1 C orange juice

     1/2 C coconut milk

     1/4 C tamari sauce

     2 T vinegar

     2 T molasses

Stir, heat slowly, and add:

     3 T cornstarch mixed in 1/4 C water

Stir and cook until thickened. Keeps well in refrigerator.

Steamed Vegetable Medley

     wax turnip/rutabaga in 5/8" cubes

     yam/sweet potato

     Brussels sprouts

     red cabbage

     red onion

     broccoli

     kale

     bell pepper

Place in steamer in order given, with bell pepper on top, and steam until tender.

Steamers come in all different sizes/shapes and forms just like people; i.e., a fold-up insert to be place in a pot, a double broiler-top pot, and a stepped pot all have holes and are used to steam/par-boil.

144

Squash Medley

Cut in half lengthwise, scoop out and discard seeds:

5 assorted squashes (butternut, acorn, large zucchini, Chinese or other squash)

For stuffing, sauté in a little canola oil:

1 large onion, diced small

1 small to medium zucchini, diced small

2 carrots, shredded

1 C peas

Mix in:

3 pts cooked brown rice

Stuff squashes and bake covered in a 400° oven for 35 - 45 minutes or until tender. Brown under broiler if desired. Remove to cool, keep warm until ready to eat.

Stuffed Zucchini Squash

Over medium low heat:

1 T canola oil & 1 T evoo

Lightly sauté:

3 shallot cloves, minced

Add and sauté:

1 C chopped celery (1/4 stalk chopped across entire stalk inc. leaves)

1/2 medium zucchini, cut into small cubes (w/skin but minus the seeds)

1/2 C finely chopped carrot (1 carrot)

Add:

2 C cooked brown rice

Mix well and let rest in pan with heat off.

Take a very large zucchini squash, cut in half lengthwise, and scoop out seeds. Stuff with rice stuffing you have just made. Bake in 350° oven until tender, approximately 35 to 40 minutes, depending on size of zucchini. If it begins to brown too much, cover with foil.

Can be baked in foil on the grill.

Variation: add chopped green beans, baby spinach, and basil to the stuffing.

Baked White Beans

Great for a morning that starts out sunny but turns cloudy.

Rinse, pick through, and soak overnight or 8 hours in a large bowl with water to cover by 2":

1/2 lb navy beans

1/2 lb small limas

Soak separately:

1/3 lb soybeans

In the morning heat over stovetop until hot in a soup pot or large Dutch oven:

2 pts vegetable broth

Cook soy beans 1 hour. Add navy beans and lima beans with water to cover by 1".
Add:

1/3 lb yellow or red split peas (do not soak)

Cook all for two hours in a 250°oven.

Add in vegetables below and cook for 1 hour additional:

first 1/3 stalk celery (with leaves), scrubbed with brush, trimmed, sliced across whole stalk

1 large carrot, diced

1 large onion, diced

Mix together:

1/2 C molasses or 1/4 C brown sugar

2 T maple syrup

2 T tomato sauce (freeze rest of can in ice cube trays, or use your own frozen cubes)

1 T mustard (dried or prepared)

Add molasses mixture to beans. Cook until all beans tender, sauce is dark and bubbly, and taste is perfect, stirring every 45 - 60 minutes for 4 - 8 hours. Serve from a bean pot if you have one, or a deep casserole dish you can keep warm.

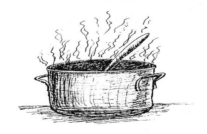

Fiber in Selected Vegetables

Food	Grams of Fiber/Serving Size	Calories/Gram of Fiber
Cabbage, steamed, boiled	10 grams/1 cup	3 calories (30 cal/serv.)
Beans, dried boiled	12 grams/1/4 cup dry 2/3 C cooked	6 calories (72 cal)
Orange	4 grams/1 orange	18 calories (72 cal)
Apple	5 grams/1 apple	23 calories (115 cal)
Bread whole grain	3+ grams/2 slices	25 calories (75 cal)
Potato boiled	2 grams/1 med. potato	79 calories (158 cal)
Bread white	< 2 grams/2 slices	87 calories (170 cal)

Why?

Why should you switch from white bread to whole grain bread?

Do you want to be part of the problem or part of the solution?

Late Winter Stir-Fry

This is the basic way to do a stir-fry. Use canola oil if you want to use a higher heat (medium high). Use olive oil for stir-frying at a lower heat (this takes longer). Extra virgin olive oil is good for salads and things that will be cooked at a very low heat. For a stir-fry, the higher the heat, the less time it takes, but the more likely it is to burn and cause carcinogens in your food, so keep the vegetables moving with a spatula. If you use high heat, cook the vegetables for just a short period of time, starting with the one that takes the longest to cook, as it will be in the skillet for the longest. Push cooked vegetables to the side and add new ones in the middle of the pan or wok.

Heat canola oil in large skillet or wok. Stir fry each of the ingredients below before adding next ingredient:

    2 carrots, sliced on diagonal
    4 radishes, sliced
    2 stalks broccoli, cut into florets

Add:

    2 T sauce, the Polynesian sauce on page 144 or the Oriental sauce on page 85
    1 T water

Stir and heat.

Optional additions:

    1/4 sweet Peruvian onion, chunked
    3 cloves garlic, smashed & sliced
    more sauce

Enjoy this slightly sweet stir-fry. Serve with brown rice.

Instead of the sauces above, you can substitute store-bought sauce from a jar or use 2 T tamari sauce.

148

Harvest Stir-Fry

Stir-fry in order given over medium high heat in a large skillet with canola oil:

fresh lima beans, removed from pods
radishes, sliced
zucchini, cubed with skin on
red pepper, diced
onion, diced
garlic, sliced
cabbage, shredded

Add a little water and cover skillet, letting vegetables steam a minute or two. Serve with tamari sauce.

Simple Stir-Fry

5-6 cauliflower florets
3 scallions
1 C peas

Stir-fry in order given. For medium high heat, use canola oil. Use lower heat with olive oil. Add tamari and pepper. Serve with brown rice.

Vegetable Stir-Fry

carrots cut on diagonal
onion in wedges 3/8" wide
celery
cauliflower
broccoli
zucchini squash
mushrooms
green pepper

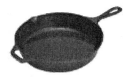

Oriental Stir-Fries

Here are some more ideas for stir-fries.

carrot
leek
baby bok choy
zucchini
napa
mushrooms
bell pepper
ginger
garlic

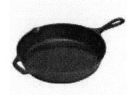

water, tamari sauce

• • •

6 broccoli buds
5 - 10 snow peas
5 - 10 kale leaves, washed & chopped
5 - 10 spinach leaves, washed & chopped
1/3 C bean sprouts

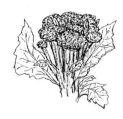

water, tamari sauce

Thicken with cornstarch and water if you want a thicker sauce.

• • •

More Oriental Stir-Fries

tofu
2 bok choy
1/4 red pepper
1 carrot
1/2 portobello mushroom
4 - 5 broccoli buds
4 - 5 snow peas

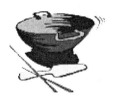

water, teriyaki sauce

•   •   •

carrot
onion
pea pods
zucchini
sliced mushrooms
asparagus
garlic & ginger

Brice's Stir-Fry

Once when red peppers were on sale and Brice needed to use up his find, he offered to do a stir-fry. Here are his ingredients. Add to skillet in order given. Method on page 148 (though he uses a lower heat and olive oil). See next page for the differences in heat and oil.

onion
garlic
cauliflower
yam
broccoli
baby zucchini squash
red peppers
Swiss chard
a little fresh mint, chopped

Special Stir-Fry

This stir-fry includes a spinach-filled sauce.

1" **ginger root,** minced
1 **clove shallot,** minced
1 **carrot,** julienne
1 **small frying pepper,** diced
1 **bunch scallions,** trimmed & cut into 1" pieces
1 **jalapeño pepper,** ends cut off, seeds removed with sharp knife, sliced into rings

1 **medium zucchini,** quartered lengthwise and sliced into 1/4" pieces
6 **crimini mushrooms,** sliced
2 **portobello mushrooms,** sliced

2 T **flour** combined with 1/2 C water
2 C **vegetable broth**

2 C **baby spinach** (about 4 handfuls)

A Word about Stir-Frying

Originally done over high heat with a high temperature fat or oil (like canola or peanut oil), the heat permeated the food pieces on the outside, and as a new item was added to the skillet (and it subsequently cooled down the pan and its ingredients), the original food pieces continued to cook on the inside.

Many people believe that stir-frying creates carcinogens and suggest lowering the temperature to medium rather than high heat, cooking for a longer period of time than traditional stir-frying. Since the Chinese and Japanese and Korean cultures have been stir-frying for many centuries, I think we need to look elsewhere for the cancer blame game. Stir-frying over high heat with canola oil is NOT done until the food is brown (and carcinogenic), but only heated, then it is pushed to the sides of the skillet or wok while another food is added to the center. Experiment yourself and see which way you like to stir-fry.

152

Stir-Fry with Rice Sticks

This stir-fry has the addition of a very thin rice noodle. I learned this method from Xiangrong Sun, a Chinese graduate student who lived at my mother's house while I was out in Iowa tending her in the early 90's. Sun cut all the vegetables up in the afternoon, leaving them to smell throughout the house and make my mother and me hungry. Then when suppertime came, she did what seemed to me an unusual way of cooking, one vegetable at a time and taking it out of the pan in between additions. Sure did taste good, though. With much patience she taught me how to make this, as the rice sticks were also new to me. You soak them in boiling hot water (use a bowl for this) for 3 - 5 minutes, then drain and rinse with cold water so they won't overcook. She used lots of rice noodles, almost like a Pad Thai recipe. I prefer a few less starchy white carbs, so I cut an 8-oz. package of rice noodles at the turn of the noodles in the package, making one package last for four recipes.

Cook vegetables one at a time in a hot skillet with canola oil, removing when very hot (slightly cooked) to a side bowl (vegetables will continue cooking when set aside). Continue in order given . Add more oil as necessary.

egg, scrambled with a little water
ginger & garlic
carrot, sliced (this can be cooked with ginger and garlic)
cauliflower, sliced
a little onion
pea pods
broccoli
zucchini
mushrooms
tomato, cut into wedges

Now add the rice sticks and all the vegetables back into the skillet, mix well, and add some **tamari sauce or soy sauce.**

A full meal to serve in a large bowl with chopsticks or a fork.

Oriental Store Shopping List

My Oriental store is huge, up on US Route 22 (a highway that cuts across central New Jersey), and it caters to restaurants. Except for being 25 miles away and having a strong fishy smell at the back of the store, it's a wonderful place to shop and spend several hours. Craig and Li Chung took the Central Jersey Vegetarian Group on a tour there and answered many of our questions about Buddhist cooking.

Chinese vegetables, esp. water spinach, Taiwanese cabbage (sweeter, not as dense) baby bok choy, soybean sprouts, ginger & other vegetables, many grown locally.

hoisin sauce
Pad Thai sauce
red curry paste
coconut milk
coconut string

egg roll wrappers, dumpling wrappers, puff pastry (frozen)

various brown rices
brown jasmine rice

dishes, bowls, pots & pans
scissors, brooms

Health Food Store Shopping List

I know some people who do all their shopping at health food stores. This will vary from place to place. Some supermarkets carry many of these items, or may be able to get them. Some health food stores carry produce, but check it for freshness. When traveling I always pick up odd and different food items when I see a health food store, adding to my staple varieties of pasta, rice, and flour.

Vicolo pizza crusts, frozen
Almond milk, original, quart boxes [wish they had small boxes!][note: they do now!]
Soy milk, original, small boxes; hemp milk
Almond butter, chunky   Other: _____
Whole wheat flour, 2 lb. bag   _____
Barley flour, oat bran   _____
Grade B maple syrup   _____

Health Food Store (cont.)

Soy margarine   _____
White cake mix, organic   _____
Hemp brownie mix, organic   _____
Various whole grain pastas   _____
Sucanat (pure dried sugar cane, with molasses content)
Olive oil, canola oil

Supplement Shopping List

Kind	Brand	Type	#	Function
Activated Quercetin w/bromelain and Vitamin C	SN	tablets	200	histamine blocker (cellular) (for allergies)
Gingko Biloba	BB	capsules	240	brain food
St. John's Wort	NW	capsules	180	mood elevator
Pau d'Arco +	NW	capsules	180	tumor inhibiter, anti-viral (South American bark)
* Astragalus +	NW	capsules	180	immune boost, anti-oxidant (root)
* Siberian Eleuthero +	NW	capsules	180	tonic (formerly Sib. Ginseng)
Hi Bio Vitamin C	Sol	tablets	200	immune booster
Vitamin E 400IU	BB	soft gels	250	blood thinner, anti-oxidant
Selenium 200 mcg	BB	tabs	300	co-metabolite/V E
CoQ10 50 mg	BB	soft gels	120	anti-oxidant
Calcium Mag Citrate	Sol	tabs	100	bone health
B Complex 50	BB	tabs	100	anti-stress
GTF Chrom. 200mcg	NOW	tabs	100	diet deficient
Chelated Manganese	Sol	tabs	100	diet deficient
Zinc Picolinate w/B6	Sol	tabs	60	diet deficient

(circled note next to last four rows: these are taken every other day)

+ I rotate these three: two on, one off, then when I run out of one, I add in the third one.

* Classified as an adaptogen, an herb that increases the body's endurance and resistance to a wide array of physical, chemical, and biological stressors. Adaptogens help normalize the functioning of various body systems by affecting the action of hormones. Adaptogens are usually beneficial in treating chronic conditions. They have been found to enhance the immune response, reduce inflammation, stabilize blood sugar, and support the hormone systems, particularly the adrenal and pituitary glands. Adaptogens should be used for an extended period of time, at least six weeks. Cannabis is also an adaptogen. — Answers.com

Note: Answers.com is based in Israel, where they have a healthy attitude about herbal remedies, and Americans are slowly changing. Hopefully seeing this chart will get others to think about herbs.

Mushroom Dinner

In a hot skillet over medium heat pour:
> 2 t canola oil
> 1 t olive oil

When hot add:
> 1 t minced ginger

Then add and stir-fry:
> 1 carrot, julienne
> 2 mushrooms, white or brown, sliced
> 1 portobello mushroom, sliced
> 1/2 onion, minced

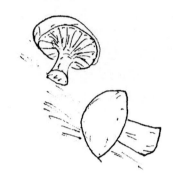

Add:
> 2 t flour

Stir and cook. Add:
> 1 C vegetable broth

Stir as it thickens. Add:
> 2 C spinach, chopped
> 1 C soy sprouts

Stir until spinach and sprouts have wilted.

Serve over brown rice.

Mushroom Dinner 2

As above:
> 3 T olive oil
> 4 shallot cloves
> 4 large portobello mushrooms
> 2 handfuls peapods, minced
> 8 green onions (scallions)
> 2 C green peas, fresh or frozen

> 2 T flour, 2 C vegetable broth (preferably clear)

> 2 C baby spinach
> 3/4 C soy sprouts

Zucchini and Garlic

First is the quick version; following is the regular stir-fry version.

Remove **garlic oil** (p.94) from refrigerator.
Get one **small zucchini** from your garden. Wash and trim ends (but do not peel).
Slice into 1/4" rounds.
Peel and slice **four cloves of garlic** (the little side pieces, not the whole bulb).
Heat **2 t extra virgin olive oil** (evoo) and **1 t garlic oil** in a small skillet over low side of medium heat (low heat keeps evoo from forming carcinogens). Sauté garlic cloves, then add squash and sauté. When squash is tender, remove and enjoy.

To stir-fry, heat small skillet over low side of high heat. Add **2 teaspoons canola oil,** quickly stir-fry the **garlic,** then the **squash.** When squash is almost done (it will continue cooking when removed from heat, so don't overdo), add **1 teaspoon garlic oil.** Stir well and remove from heat. Enjoy this cleansing lunch (or breakfast).

Cravings

When you get a craving, when your body tells you you need something, it simply means you're out of balance, usually from bad diet or stress hormones. Imbalance can show itself as odd itching (I once had a doctor I dated tell me this was the brain "misfiring"), a chill you get when you take a step, a twinge of pain from your shoulder.

If you step in early, watching yourself on a daily basis, you can avoid the terrible depression surges, anger surges, withdrawal surges, and food cravings. You can do a variety of things to right this imbalance, no matter what the cause. A slight imbalance could just be a sign of impending disease. It is your choice how to right this imbalance.
Things some people do:
1) wallow in it
2) eat sugary or starchy (candy bar or French fries) or overly processed food
3) sleep (here at least the body has a chance to balance itself through restorative sleep)
4) watch TV (flip around until something grabs your attention, then veg until you feel better)

My suggestions:
Drink water (dilutes the blood), intentional breathing (oxygenates the brain), meditate, go for a walk or do yoga stretches (helps redistribute toxins, oxygenate blood, esp. in brain).

And eat a better balanced diet tomorrow.

Almond, Soy, and Hemp Milk Nutrients

	Almond Milk	Soy Milk	Hemp Milk
Amount	1 C	1 C	1 C
Calories	90 cal	135 cal	110 cal
Fat	2.5 gms	5 gms	7 gms
Carbs	15 gms	14 gms	7 gms
Protein	2 gms	10 gms	5 gms
Fiber	1 gm	1 gm	1 gm
Sugar	9 gms	7 gms	6 gms
Calcium	2% MDR	8% MDR	2% MDR
Iron	6% MDR	10% MDR	20% MDR

Almond milk has less fat and fewer calories.
Soy milk has more calcium, iron, and protein.
Hemp milk has even more iron, more fat, and fewer carbs.
Some items above vary from manufacturer to manufacturer.

Green Bean Dinner

Wash, remove ends, and split in two lengthwise if large (leave whole if not):

1 pound green beans

Steam over boiling water in steamer for 5 minutes. Cool. This can be done early in the day, as is done in Chinese restaurants.

To stir-fry, heat in skillet over medium hot heat:

1 T canola oil

Add and stir-fry:

2 cloves garlic, sliced

1 large onion, chopped

Add to skillet and stir-fry:

4 regular mushrooms, sliced

1 small zucchini, sliced

At end stir-fry:

prepared green beans

Add a little tamari sauce and/or water, put a lid on skillet, and let steam for 2 minutes. Remove lid and stir.

Serve over brown rice.

Working Supper

If you are having great difficulty getting rid of fried foods.

Heat:

1 t olive oil

Add:

2 small red potatoes, diced

1 carrot, diced

1 onion, diced

4 mushrooms, sliced

1 stalk broccoli, broken into florets

Cover and steam over low heat until broccoli is tender enough to eat.

Onions

All my life I used yellow onions. I never used that much at a time as they were so strong. Then I met a man I began to cook for, and he *loved* onions. So I increased the amount of yellow onions I used.

Then one time in 2002 a young chef I knew asked me if I had ever used Vidalia onions. *No, I hadn't.* On his suggestion I tried one, in season (early spring through the summer), and liked them MUCH better than yellow onions. They weren't so strong, but they still had that onion flavor.

Most Vidalia onions are large, making them easier to handle, slice, and dice. Now that they have figured out how to extend the life of the Vidalia onion (storing dry at 92% nitrogen, 3% oxygen) they don't peter out in the middle of the summer, but we can get them through the end of the year, making them great for late summer and fall cooking.

I also found that very thin slices of Vidalia onion are perfect for keeping the lettuce and spinach fresh in a salad if they are layered directly on top of the greens. I put a layer of shredded carrots on top of the onion, as carrots will also deteriorate when shredded, but the onion serves as an anti-biotic to keep them crisp and tasty.

I have moved beyond these two onions, also, and tried shallots, green onions (scallions), and purple onions, each of which has its own season. Get to know your produce person, and they will point out which onions are the freshest and in season. You can substitute what is freshest if you don't have or can't find what I suggest.

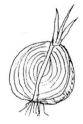  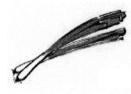

Sweet and Sour Vegetables

Add to large skillet or wok and stir-fry in order given in a little canola oil:

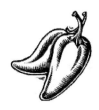

1 carrot, sliced at an angle
1 jalapeño pepper, diced or sliced
1 medium Vidalia onion, diced
1 stalk celery, chopped
4 mushrooms, sliced
1 large red pepper, large dice
1 regular tomato, cut in half, then into wedges
5 cloves garlic, smashed & sliced
24 pineapple cubes (2 slices)

Stir in a mixture of:

1/2 C water
1/2 C pineapple juice
1/3 C Sucanat or brown sugar
2 T vinegar
1/4 C potato flakes (1 T cornstarch)

Stir and cook until thickened. Adjust seasonings and serve over brown rice.

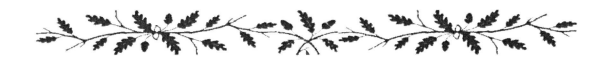

Afterthoughts

Whew! It's finished!

By now I hope you've stopped thinking of food as just something you buy at the supermarket and you've started thinking of it as life energy that you put into your body. Following the seasons is one way of connecting with nature. Food is the key to that connection between you and "the nourishment stream." Thinking about your food in this way points you towards, reintegrates you with, *qi*, with *gaia* (mother earth), with god. You get your nourishment from that connection, that energy flow, that love. These ideas are not new, but are ancient.

I want to thank Stacey of the Central Jersey Vegetarian Group for her steadfast adherence to her beliefs in the rights of animals, to the exclusion of many foods I consider irrefutable. She has been a good role-model for me, along with other members of the group. More information on CJVG may be found at www.cjvg.org.

I also want to acknowledge my indebtedness to Irma Rombauer, author of *Joy of Cooking,* with the biography of her that follows mine. I understand it was written by her daughter, and appears in current editions of the cookbook.

It is an absolute miracle that some of the recipes, written on a Mac in 2001, went through 3 PCs and two laptops, Windows 98 and Windows XP, many e-mails, two more PCs, and several flash drives, plus the printer's computers, before they landed on the pages in the book you hold. I figure there must be some unknown reason the knowledge in this book was able to come through all that technology, and that I was given the patience to help it through.

Sally Miller

May 2009

Sally Miller

Sally Miller grew up in the Midwest on the campus of Iowa State, home of one of the finest home economics schools in the country. Her parents were Southerners (from Oklahoma) of German heritage, and though both cooked, most of the domestic food preparation fell on Sally's mother. Sally's father, an engineer, designed the kitchen in their home (now the Women's Center at ISU) to be comfortable and efficient for the whole family, especially for Sally's mother, who was only five feet tall.

Sally thought all young women were schooled in cooking as she and her two sisters had been, but her education was truly unique. Besides Sally having parents who cooked, home-ec "student girls" who lived at their house — working for room and board while in school at Iowa State — frequently brought their classwork home to the family.

One running family joke: At dinner Sally's father would pick up one of the muffins a student had just made in practicing for her next-day cooking class. He'd turn it around, slowly break it open, and carefully examine the air holes within the muffin. Eventually he would proclaim, *I don't think this is standard product!* much to the embarrassment of the crestfallen student. Then the family members would all laugh, tell her how good the muffins tasted, and rib her a little more to make her feel comfortable again.

Sally's more formal cooking education began with classes at Iowa State in the late 1950's and continued in the late 60's and 70's at Rutgers University in New Brunswick NJ, which had a good home-economics department in its own right. By that time she was fixing meals for a family of six. One paper she wrote for a home-ec class featured a cook-ahead meal for company which came out of the freezer, foreshadowing many meals to come.

Eventually Sally fell into the habit many Americans fall into, buying and eating food fixed by others, either from the supermarket freezer case or at a restaurant. However, after her operation for ovarian cancer in 1996, rather than use the conventional treatments of chemotherapy or radiation, she began to look at food in a new way — a way that would allow her body to heal naturally and be supported with the nutrition she needed to be healthy. She joined the Central Jersey Vegetarian Group, where animal rights, religious, ethical, and health-conscious vegetarians met for support, education, and social networking. Along with her son Dave she became co-chair of the Restaurant Committee, which selected various restaurants where members could dine. Indian, Mexican, Ethiopian, Chinese, Thai, Spanish, Buddhist, raw food, and vegan restaurants provided many new dishes to try. These experiences influenced Sally's personal cooking, and she, in turn, shared her new knowledge with others through cooking classes, private consultations, and a 2001 cookbook *Good Eats at Sally's,* which contains health and nutritional information in addition to recipes.

Sally's in the Kitchen, Sally Miller's second cookbook, features a variety of ethnic, plant-based, and large-volume recipes to freeze for future use, especially handy for health conscious working people and those who run home-based businesses. Regional dishes and personal family favorites round out the 200-page volume.

Irma Rombauer

Irma von Starkloff Rombauer (1877 - 1962), a Missouri homemaker who developed "The Joy of Cooking" at the age of 54, is one of the most influential figures in American home cooking in the twentieth century. "The Joy of Cooking" has been continuously in print since 1936.

A Privileged Upbringing

The youngest child of a well-off St. Louis doctor, Max von Starkloff and his second wife Emma Kuhlmann, Rombauer was born October 30, 1877. The Starkloff family lived in Carondelet, a former suburb of St. Louis, which had been annexed by the city less than a decade before Rombauer's birth. During her early childhood, Rombauer and her elder sister, Elsa, were educated at home and later at local schools. When Rombauer was twelve, her father took a government posting in Bremen, Germany, where the family remained for five years. During these years, she continued her somewhat sporadic formal education, being taught by governesses or at girls' schools in Bremen or, briefly, Lausanne. In late summer 1894, the von Starkloffs returned to Missouri, settling in fashionable South St. Louis.

Upon the family's return, Rombauer began taking art courses at local Washington University - although she did not formally pursue a degree - and spent time visiting family in Indianapolis. In 1897, the still-Irma von Starkloff met young lawyer Edgar Rombauer; the two became engaged in early 1899 and married in a civil ceremony on October 14 of that year. Rombauer's income was limited, and the young couple lived in a small rented apartment with reportedly no domestic help, a state which Anne Mendelson noted in *Stand Facing the Stove* was "outlandish indeed for a bride of [Rombauer's] social position," adding that this story may have been an exaggeration.

Married Life

Short months after the Rombauers' marriage, the couple's first child, Roland, was born on July 27, 1900. However, the baby was not strong and died in March of the following year. Both father and mother were devastated by this loss, and the Rombauers left their apartment to move in with the von Starkloffs. In March 1902, Edgar Rombauer had a nervous breakdown; to help him recover, he and his wife traveled to a resort at Eureka Springs, Arkansas. By the end of April, he was sufficiently recovered to return to St. Louis, where the couple's second child and only daughter, Marion, was born on January 2, 1903. The growing family continued to live with the von Starkloffs until 1906, when Edgar Rombauer became the legal guardian of his fourteen-year-old nephew, Roderick, and the Rombauers took up residence in the home of their new charge's deceased family. (Roderick, who turned out to be a somewhat rebellious and unruly teenager, quickly found himself sent to military school.)

The Rombauer family grew in a more traditional way the following year, when Irma Rombauer gave birth to what would be the last Rombauer child, Edgar Roderick Rombauer Junior, on August 15, 1907. Rombauer was not a traditional mother figure, spending much of her time out of the house; after 1911, she was particularly involved with St. Louis' elite Wednesday Club. Edgar Rombauer was an avid outdoorsman, and the family maintained a vacation cottage in Michigan. Here, Rombauer would later claim, she learned the basics of cooking from her husband. As the Rombauer children progressed through school and their parents through their upper-middle-class lives, nothing portended that Irma Rombauer would, in middle age, write one of America's most enduring cookbooks.

Tragedy Spurred *The Joy of Cooking*

By 1929, Irma Rombauer had become prominent in St. Louis' social circles, serving that year, for example, as president of the Women's Committee of the St. Louis Symphony Orchestra Board of Directors. However, her husband had continued to suffer nervous attacks every few years since the initial breakdown in 1902; in the fall of 1929, a particularly severe breakdown struck him. Mendelson comments that "despite the timing, it is doubtful that the Great Depression ... was the clue to this collapse." Possibly contributing factors included a recent loss in a Board of Education election or a possible recurrence of a bladder cancer Edgar Rombauer had battled years previously. Whatever the cause, the Rombauers spent most of December 1929 and January 1930 in South Carolina in the hopes that the milder climate would ease Rombauer's recovery. When the couple returned to St. Louis at the end of January, Edgar Rombauer seemed improved and ready to return to normal life.

However, on February 3, 1930, while Irma Rombauer was out of the house shopping, Edgar Rombauer committed suicide by shooting himself through the mouth with a shotgun. The act was completely unexpected and the Rombauer family was shocked and devastated. To complicate matters, the Great Depression was taking its toll on Irma Rombauer; she realized quickly that she would need to find another source of income to replace the money her husband had earned. Rombauer moved to a smaller, cheaper apartment in the West End of St. Louis. Unable to fathom the idea of finding regular employment, she determined to write a cookbook to bring in some money.

An Amateur Wrote a Classic

No evidence of Rombauer having any experience or talent as a cook exists. Rather than using her own recipes exclusively, Rombauer spent months collecting recipes from acquaintances, testing them to decide whether or not they would suitable for inclusion in her burgeoning cookbook. Her daughter Marion, then living in New York City, assisted in the testing process and later, illustrated the manuscript. Rombauer did not have a publisher for the cook-book, instead used part of her $6,000 legacy from her husband's death to pay the Clayton Company to print 3,000 copies of *The Joy of Cooking: a Compilation of Reliable Recipes with a Casual Culinary Chat*. Indeed, to fans of the cookbook, much of its charm lies in Rombauer's chatty tone, with anecdotes woven into the recipes. Unlike traditional cookbooks, Rombauer's voice infuses *The Joy of Cooking*, as though she were sitting in the kitchen of each reader, telling them personally how to prepare a certain dish. Rombauer marketed the book herself, selling copies to friends; convincing shops in St. Louis, Michigan, and other areas to carry the cookbook; and generating publicity through contacts with newspapers.

The original release of *The Joy of Cooking* enjoyed modest success. In *Little Acorn*, Irma Rombauer's daughter Marion Rombauer Becker commented that "Mother's friends made sales lively, but not brisk enough to suit her." By 1935, an expanded version was set to be published by Bobbs-Merrill. Rombauer and her publisher had an acrimonious relationship from the start, often arguing over costs and royalties. However, when the cookbook was released nationally in 1936, it enjoyed moderate success and seemed to be on its way to becoming a standard, accepted cookbook like the popular *Fannie Farmer's Boston Cooking-School Cookbook*. The 1936 edition introduced what was then a revolutionary format for the recipes themselves; instead of listing the ingredients directly after the recipe's title and then providing instructions for the creation of the dish, *The Joy of Cooking* presented the directions chronologically, setting the required ingredients in bold type.

Rombauer Chose an Heir

By the mid-1940s, when *The Joy of Cooking* truly became an unmitigated success, Irma Rombauer was approaching her 70th birthday. Her health was starting to fade, perhaps spurred by her stressful working relationship with her publisher and some family disputes. Rombauer's next cookbook, *A Cookbook for Girls and Boys*, was completed with the assistance of her daughter Marion Rombauer Becker, by then living in Cincinnati, Ohio. Although Rombauer Becker had provided mostly artistic contributions to previous editions, the 1951 revision of *The Joy of Cooking* recognized her as a genuine co-author. She, rather than her mother, took up much of the debate with Bobbs-Merrill over matters related to the publication of the cookbook, only truly taking over as head of the content later.

With the 1951 edition safely handled, Irma Rombauer, indulging a life-long love of travel, set off to Europe with her grandson for an extended tour and later visited Mexico City. However, in 1955, at 78, she suffered a mild stroke; although this stroke did not impair her mental process, it did mark the beginning of a continuing series of strokes that struck Rombauer down over the next few years. These strokes gradually robbed Rombauer of her strength, speech, and ability to perform even simple tasks such as writing. She found herself in a situation she had feared: being unable to control her body, while maintaining mental awareness and her sense of self. Marion Rombauer Becker was forced to take control of *The Joy of Cooking* due to her mother's deteriorating health.

Rombauer's health continued to falter and, in 1962, at last failed. Her first stroke had paralyzed the left side of her body; now, her left leg had become infected with gangrene. To complicate the problem, Rombauer had an irregular heartbeat and had recently experienced a bout of seizures triggered by the failure of some brain functions. Her left leg was amputated but did not properly heal. Rombauer was transferred to a nursing home due to the infection from her leg and died there after a steady deterioration on October 17, 1962.

The Later History of *The Joy of Cooking*

After her mother's death, Marion Rombauer Becker became responsible for the updates and revisions to *The Joy of Cooking* until the mid-1970s. The cookbook then remained essentially unchanged for nearly two decades, with her fifth edition acting as the standard text. In 1997, Ethan Becker, Marion Rombauer Becker's son and Irma Rombauer's grandson, headed up a major revision, incorporating more modern recipes and ingredients. The following year, Ethan Becker wrote an introduction for Simon and Schuster's reprint of an exact reproduction of the original 1931 self-published edition with Marion Rombauer Becker's illustrations. *The Joy of Cooking* today remains one of the most respected cookbooks in America, considered by many to be one of the most essential cooking texts available.

Biography from Answers.com

Groupings

6. Salads

Cabbage Tuna Salad *	138
Carrot Spinach Salad	138
Chicken Salad *	131
Cinco de Mayo Salad	121
DaveFest Drizzle	32
Fruity Salads	133
Garden Salad	21
Hot Cucumber Salad	15
Picnic Bean Salad	6
Pico de Gallo	7
Quick Pix	14
Quick Salads	10
Raggedy Ann Salad *	24
Salad Rap	138
Salad Wrap	21
Tex-Mex Bean Salad	10
Tuna Macaroni Salad *	11
Winter Salad	83

7. Sandwiches, Spreads, and Snacks

Black Olive Spread	67
Bruschetta	12
Garlic Oil	94
Hinky Dink *	1
Mexican Buns *	9
Mushroom Hot Wrap	67
Perfect Veggie Burger	9
Puffs	106-107
Quick Bruschetta	139
Roasted Pecans	70
Seven-Layer Sandwich *	25
Summer Sandwich	139
Tostitos Casserole *	52
Winter Bruschetta	88

> * Items with an asterisk contain meat, eggs, and/or dairy as a significant part of the recipe or menu. Others that contain eggs or dairy can remain essentially the same with substitutes or by leaving non-vegan item out.

8. Soups and Drinks

Butternut Squash Soup	141
Cabbage Soup	141
Carrot Soup	32
Christmas Soup *	142
Coffee Tea	109
Fall Breakfast Drink	139
Fruit Drink	3
Green Bean Chowder	142
Hot and Sour Soup	93
Mushroom Barley Soup	66
Onion Soup	140
Orange Mint Drink	2
Potato Cauliflower Soups	62
Reefer Soup	40
Southern Soup	45
Tomato Barley Soup	46
Vegetable Pea Soup	140
Zen Iced Tea	133

9. Toppings, Sauces, Gravy, Stuffing

Apricot Scallion Sesame Sauce	85
Cranberry Sauce	52
Cucumbers and Cream *	14
Crumbs	18
Lentil Gravy	51
Lime Butter Sauce	130
Pizza Sauce	143
Polynesian Sauce	144
Puff Sauce	107
Rice Stuffing	31
Turkey Gravy *	55
Turkey Stuffing *	54

10. Vegetables: Baked, Steamed, Boiled

Baked White Beans	146
Baked Vegetables	65
Boiled Dinner	96
Broccoli with Garlic Sauce	108
Butternut Squash Rounds	31
Cauliflower Au Gratin	137
Chili Mac *	125
Chinese New Year	84
Enchiladas *	121

11. Vegetables: Fried, Stir-Fried

12. Volume Cooking and Preserving

13. X-tras

> * Items with an asterisk contain meat, eggs, and/or dairy as a significant part of the recipe or menu and would not be suitable for vegans. Others that contain eggs or dairy remain essentially the same with substitutes or by leaving non-vegan item out.

Alphabetical Index

> * Items with an asterisk contain meat, eggs, and/or dairy as a significant part of the recipe or menu.

* Items with an asterisk contain meat, eggs, and/or dairy as a significant part of the recipe or menu and would not be suitable for vegans. Others that contain eggs or dairy can remain essentially the same with substitutes or by leaving non-vegan item out.

Synergy Books

All books by Sally Miller unless otherwise noted

Jersey Girl Fantasies	$15
Family Affair Fantasies	$20
Enema Fantasies	$20
Animal Fantasies	$20
Fantasies of the Future	$20
Bloomers (a novel by Gregor Samsa)	$20
Hunterdon Girl Fantasies	$20
Hair (readers)	$20
Synergy Reader (readers)	$20
Enema Memories (readers)	$20
ABC's of Living Without Cancer	$20
Good Eats At Sally's (cookbook)	$20
Sylvia, A Memoir of Hollywood Star Sylvia Sidney	$15
Times Queer (Mykola Dementiuk)	$15
Times Queer (e-book with pictures)	$5
Baby Doll (Mykola Dementiuk)	$12
Selected Tales (Mykola Dementiuk)	$13
Vienna Dolorosa (a novel by Mykola Dementiuk)	$25
Holy Communion (a novel by Mykola Dementiuk)	$25
Sally's in the Kitchen (cookbook)	$25
The Truth According to Sally Miller (essays) 2009	$25
100 Whores (Mykola Dementiuk) 2009	$25

Any three books, $50
Times Queer E-book free with $100 order (include e-mail address)

All prices include Media postage
Add $2 for Canadian/Mexican orders, $5 ROW

Synergy Book Service, POB 8, Flemington NJ 08822
(908) 782-7101
Synergy@SynergyBookService.com

For further details on books:
SynergyBookService.com
SylviaTheBook.com
ViennaDolorosa.com
HolyCommunionANovel.com